Growing Up with Languages

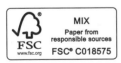

MIX
Paper from
responsible sources
FSC® C018575

PARENTS' AND TEACHERS' GUIDES

Series Editor: Colin Baker, *Bangor University, UK*

This series provides immediate advice and practical help on topics where parents and teachers frequently seek answers. Each book is written by one or more experts in a style that is highly readable, non-technical and comprehensive. No prior knowledge is assumed: a thorough understanding of a topic is promised after reading the appropriate book.

Full details of all the books in this series and of all our other publications can be found on http://www.multilingual-matters.com, or by writing to Multilingual Matters, St Nicholas House, 31–34 High Street, Bristol BS1 2AW, UK.

Growing Up with Languages

Reflections on Multilingual Childhoods

Claire Thomas

MULTILINGUAL MATTERS
Bristol • Buffalo • Toronto

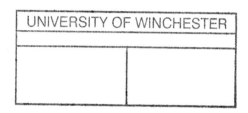
Library of Congress Cataloging in Publication Data
A catalog record for this book is available from the Library of Congress.
Thomas, Claire.
Growing up with Languages: Reflections on Multilingual Childhoods/Claire Thomas.
Parents' and Teachers' Guides: 15
Includes bibliographical references and index.
1. Multilingualism in children. 2. Parenting. 3. Children--Language. 4. Families--Language. I. Title.
P115.2.T56 2012
404'.2083–dc23 2012009125

British Library Cataloguing in Publication Data
A catalogue entry for this book is available from the British Library.

ISBN-13: 978-1-84769-715-8 (hbk)
ISBN-13: 978-1-84769-714-1 (pbk)

Multilingual Matters
UK: St Nicholas House, 31–34 High Street, Bristol BS1 2AW, UK.
USA: UTP, 2250 Military Road, Tonawanda, NY 14150, USA.
Canada: UTP, 5201 Dufferin Street, North York, Ontario M3H 5T8, Canada.

The policy of Multilingual Matters/Channel View Publications is to use papers that are natural, renewable and recyclable products, made from wood grown in sustainable forests. In the manufacturing process of our books, and to further support our policy, preference is given to printers that have FSC and PEFC Chain of Custody certification. The FSC and/or PEFC logos will appear on those books where full certification has been granted to the printer concerned.

Typeset by The Charlesworth Group.
Printed and bound in Great Britain by the MPG Books Group.

Contents

Acknowledgements

All of us at Waltham Forest Bilingual Group (WFBG) are very grateful to the very many people and organisations that have helped the team carry out this research and I am personally grateful to all those who have supported me whilst I analysed and wrote this book.

Firstly, to all the interviewees who shared their memories with us, we appreciate that for many of you, we asked you to think about and share things in a way that you may have never done before. We particularly appreciate those who shared sad or more difficult memories and experiences with us.

To the interview team: Bettina Coleman Schoels, Didier Cordina, Mirela Dumic, and Ulrike Rűb-Taylor.

For contacting potential interviewees: Cecile Clerc, Anne Gaskell, Ricky Lowes, Isabelle Merminod, Davina Thomas, and Multilingual Families magazine.

To Ricky Lowes (without her WFBG would not exist) and to all those who have helped run WFBG since its creation, particularly Chris and Didier Cordina and Karin Laumann.

For providing comments on the draft text Bettina Coleman Schoels, Chris Cordina, Claudia Williams, Colin Baker, Didier Cordina, Jean-Marc Dewaele, John Williams, Mirela Dumic, Ricky Lowes, Shahnaz Qizilbash, Snjezana Bokulic, and Ulrike Rűb-Taylor.

To Choni Barrio and her family for the cover photo.

For providing funding for the interviews – The National Lottery Awards for All.

For providing funding for the ongoing work of WFBG, the Esmée Fairbairn Foundation.

For giving me time off work to write up part of the book, Minority Rights Group International.

For caring for my children, so I could carve out more writing time, Chris Carlsson and Starr and Colin Thomas.

For his kind, thoughtful, and helpful advice, Colin Baker.

Finally, of course, to my bilingual children, Renee and Olivier, and their father, Jean-Marie.

Introduction

This book opens a window into the minds of children in multilingual families. Uniquely, we interviewed adults who had been raised speaking more than one language and asked them to share their experiences with us. Many books have been written based on interviews with *parents* in multilingual families as to their views of what has worked or not from their point of view. But the parents can only guess what their children are thinking and feeling. We believe many parents will find it useful to get this insight into multilingual children's lives.

When Colin Baker (a leading authority on multilingualism in the UK) came to talk to our group, he told us:

'When your children are grown up, they will be glad that you made the effort to raise them bilingually'.

To test out this statement, we asked adults a wide range of questions about their multilingual childhoods. We were lucky that many of them had excellent memories and shared their recollections with us – some were happier and more successful in their multilingualism than others. Interviewees expressed, at times, resentment, resistance, and subtle regrets. However, ultimately they all – without exception – proved Colin Baker right.

This was important to us, as we have repeated this to parents in our group who have concerns or who may be tempted to give up when times are tough. We repeated the phrase, but more as a mantra than anything else until we got round to asking the question, 'Is there evidence backing it? Have books been written collecting the views of people, now adult, about their multilingual childhoods?' The answer was no. If the bald statement is encouraging for parents when it is essentially taken on trust, how much more convincing and useful would be detailed accounts from adults stating how they feel as adults, but also telling us how it felt to be bilingual and growing up. This was the starting point for this book. We are a group of multilingual families and we felt that evidence backing up the 'they will thank you when they're grown up' statement would help us understand how things felt from our children's point of view and help us to decide which strategies to use and when. The book covers most, if not all, of the common dilemmas, decisions, and problems which parents in multilingual families encounter. It is based on over 40 detailed interviews with adults who had grown up on different continents, speaking widely different languages and with a huge variety of environments, experiences and circumstances.

The interviewing team and myself are all active members of a small self-help group of parents raising children bilingually. We meet once a month to discuss issues that we are facing, concerns we have and to share tips and experiences. This means that we are all aware of many of the questions commonly asked by parents and the issues that arise in families raising children multilingually. This background knowledge of what concerns parents informed the interviews and our analysis of the material.

This book is primarily aimed at parents who are raising children bilingually or multilingually. Academics and students will also find lots of interest here and many teachers will be interested in Chapter 6.

I hope that this book will help those bringing up children bilingually in several ways. Firstly, I hope that new parents will read it when they are deciding what languages to speak with their new baby. Patterns once established can be surprisingly hard to change. It is worth thinking things through fully at the outset to try to make the best decisions – to start as you mean to go on.

I hope that parents will remember the book when their children are resisting or making little or no progress in one or other language (or even both) and they are tempted to give up on the whole project. I hope that parents will also read and remember it when they are given misleading and inaccurate advice by well-meaning relatives or professionals.

Many parents of bilingual children wonder (or at times, worry) about what is going through their children's heads. This book might provide some insight by telling the stories of other similar children having similar experiences (in fact those experiences are recalled by adults who look back on their childhood experiences with some perspective).

However, those looking for 'off the shelf' solutions, or easy and straightforward answers to complex questions, will not find them here. Actually, we do not believe that 'off the shelf solutions' or simple answers are often of much help to parents in multilingual families. There are too many variables, and even situations that might seem quite similar will involve nuances and personalities that might mean that things work very differently in practice. Families are intensely personal, and what works for one family may not work for another. What this book is more likely to provide is forewarning of issues and concerns, so that parents may be able to recognise them early. Forewarning is more significant than it may sound. It may allow parents to react more quickly and appropriately than if they have to work out every issue from first principles each time it arises. Sometimes decisions need to be made in advance of any experience at all (about language use in the family when a first baby is born, about potential moves, about educational options) and this book may help parents to make more informed choices in these situations. Although we do not supply simple solutions, what parents will find is a range of options or strategies that they can pick and choose from to suit their own situation.

Children are also different. Some are simply better at picking up language than others. They have different personalities. In this book we have pitched our advice somewhat cautiously, at most with the average child in mind. So, for example, if we say, 'don't assume children will retain a language that they speak before they move to a new country. However fluently they speak it when they move, they will lose it very quickly unless they get significant continued input', this does not mean that some exceptional children would not be able to retain a language with very limited input after such a move, and there are several examples of those that did in this book – Astrid (p.31), Christine (p.57) and Fatima (p.43). However, you would not be wise to bank or plan for this. Conversely, if your child has learning difficulties or a disability, although many of the principles will be the same, we suggest that you get very specialist help and support about bilingualism.

One direct and unavoidable consequence of the decision to interview adults about their childhoods is that this book is discussing events of a few years ago. There are some differences in the context for children today compared to our interviewees, but many other aspects of bilingual family life 10, 20, 30 or more years ago remain the same. The most obvious changes are developments in communication and the media, particularly the internet and satellite TV, as well as probably a diminishing level of racism in many places and some progress in minority language policies (e.g. in Wales, the Basque country and for Spanish speakers in the United States). But there are also subtler differences; for example, our sample of mixed-language relationships included only relationships between those who spoke different European languages, whereas children growing up bilingually today in mixed language families in the UK or Europe are much more likely to speak one Asian or African language and one European language, and to be mixed race children as well as having different linguistic heritages. Another example is that although we did interview six people affected by divorce during their childhoods, in none of these were children in a joint or shared custody arrangement. Ideally we would have liked to include a child who spent half the week in one house with one parent speaking one language, and half the week in another house speaking another language with another parent. These arrangements were much less common a few decades ago.

As a result of these limitations, the book will not touch on every aspect that may concern a modern bilingual family. However, overall most parents raising children bilingually today will find a family with many similar characteristics to their own family in this book. Migrants to the UK today face many of the same issues as migrants did 30 years ago. There are just as many mixed-language families now (if not more) and the experiences of similar families some years ago still have direct relevance today.

Although many of our interviewees spoke various languages at different points of their childhoods, some lost these languages when the input ceased. Nonetheless, no less than 14 of our interviewees reached adulthood with an ability to speak three or four languages. This came about in a wide variety of different ways: children were in a bilingual home with an additional language from school, children were in bilingual homes and learnt a third language from the community, or children were in homes where three languages were spoken. Two of our interviewees were quadrilingual – one, whose parents each spoke one language, spent a considerable amount of time with a godmother who spoke a third and was taught in a fourth language at school, while the other spoke Farsi at home, and lived in France, England and Sweden whilst she was growing up. I have not devoted a separate chapter to interviewees who are trilingual or quadrilingual as the issues that arose in interviews were broadly the same regardless of how many languages were involved, whether two, three, four or even more.

We routinely tell parents in our workshops that every bilingual family is different, and those interviewed for this book proved this point if no other. Not only are they all different, but the cross-cutting, overlapping and intersecting issues make it very hard to divide up the interviewees and the issues that they raised in any way that makes total sense. For convenience, however, the 43 interviewees can be divided into four groups: those who had two or more languages spoken at home, those who spoke one language at home and another in the community and school, those who were bilingual solely through attending school in another language and those who had learnt a language solely through interacting with the community, and the specific issues within these groups are discussed in Part 1, Chapters 1–4. Here I also discuss smaller numbers of interviewees who experienced major changes during their bilingual childhoods, as a result of divorce (Chapter 5), the death of a parent (Chapter 6), as a result of advice given to parents (Chapter 7) and as a result of the interviewees own decisions or choices (Chapter 8). Part 2 discusses a range of factors which arise for all families no matter of what type, ranging from consistency or flexibility in language rules at home (Chapter 9), encouragement, rewards and sanctions (Chapter 10), children resisting their parents' wishes (Chapter 11), interviewees who felt that they stood out or did not fit in (Chapter 12) and other input from relatives, books, films, and holidays (Chapter 13). Part 3 explores the complex area of education for multilingual children. This includes starting school in a language you do not understand or speak fluently and moving schools (Chapter 14), support for home languages in mainstream schools (Chapter 15), additional forms of support outside school – mainly Saturday schools (Chapter 16), and help with homework (Chapter 17).

Part 4 looks at factors that are more external to the family – the status of different languages, racism and the impact on our families of language policies and politics.

Part 5 covers the interviewees as adults, including their views on any advantages or disadvantages of bilingualism and what advice they would pass on to a family just starting out. Facets of adult life covered include relationships, accents, learning additional languages and feelings about identity, as well as the decisions interviewees had taken about raising their own children monolingually or multilingually.

The final section of the book, Part 6, analyses which factors seemed to be linked with successful or unsuccessful outcomes and pulls together a set of recommendations for parents based on the interviews tempered with our experience of talking to many parents during the running of the WFBG group.

How to Get the Most Out of This Book

How you read this book will depend on how much time you have and what stage you and your family are at or interested in. If you are very early on in your multilingual family life, then I would strongly suggest that you read either Chapter 1 if you are in a mixed-language family, or Chapter 2 if you use one language at home but another outside the home. Most parents in most multilingual families will find some useful material in Part 2, which discusses many decisions and dilemmas that are common to all different types of family and which affect most of us at one time or another. Chapters 5–7 include many issues that you may hope will never apply to you (such as divorce or the death of a parent). But they do also include some heart warming and inspiring examples of children taking matters into their own hands, which are instructive for all parents. Very importantly, these chapters also include some example of families who changed the languages that they spoke to their children as a result of advice they received from those outside the family – cautionary tales – and everyone should read Chapter 7.

If your children are over the age of about seven, if you do not have much time, and you have a particular concern, for example, linked to schooling, you could just read an individual section or chapter, such as Part 3, or a chapter on a specific topic (e.g. on childcare or grandparents). However, if you do this you will risk missing a particular tip or strategy which may never have occurred to you, but which could still be useful.

Part 5 is for all those who would like to try to see into the future as it tells us what the interviewees are doing as adults. So it is not to be missed!

If you are very pressed for time, it is possible to just skip to Chapters 29 and 30 (on factors linked to success or failure, interviewees' advice to parents and our recommendations to parents respectively). However, if you do so you will have to take on trust how we have reached these conclusions and the particular settings and circumstances that they emerged in. Given that every family is different, this may not be the wisest course. However, one option would be to read the recommendations first and then go back and read the evidence and analysis that leads up to them and which backs them up.

Whatever other parts of the book you decide to read, I would strongly advise that you do read Chapters 29 and 30. Although there are summaries and conclusions throughout the book, Chapter 30 is where we pull together the myriad lessons from all the other sections in a way intended to be practically useful to parents.

Throughout the book, quotes of what an interviewee actually said are in *italics*. If you feel that a particular interviewee's story seems to be particularly relevant to your situation and you would like to read the interview summary in full, the full text of all the interview summaries can be found at www.wfbilingual.org.

I have avoided using any technical terms in this book but if you are unsure about what something means there is a glossary of terms (pp. 243–244).

Interviews – Key Facts at a Glance

Some interviewees preferred to remain anonymous and, in these cases, names have been changed. Throughout the book I will refer to particular individuals on several occasions where their experiences or memories are relevant. The first time that I mention a particular interviewee I will summarise the key facts about where they lived and the languages that they spoke. However, I do not necessarily repeat this each and every time that person is mentioned (as this becomes very repetitive). So here is a list of all the interviewees by name, together with the essential facts about their situations.

If I refer to someone and you need to jog your memory about the languages they spoke or their situation, you should be able to quickly refer to this table and look up the information you need (the index at the end of the book also lists each time an interviewee is referred to or quoted).

Name	Languages used as a child	As a child lived in	Particular issues arising
Adeyinka	English, Yoruba	Nigeria	Yoruba (dialects) at home and in the community, English at school. English as high prestige language.
Aimee	French, Kabye, Mina	Togo, France	Trilingual as a young girl through school and community, effect of parents' divorce as she moved to France to live with her aunt. Loss of one language through lack of input.
Antony	English, Greek	UK	Two Greek parents. Siblings spoke in English, which parents did not understand. Father tried to change this but failed. Negative about language school.
Armelle	French, Spanish	Spain, France, Argentina, Italy	French father, Spanish mother. Bilingual relationship between parents, resisted replying to her mother in French, less supportive grandparents, choosing where to live as an adult.
Astrid	English, German	Australia, Germany (briefly)	Two German parents who spoke to her in English. Bilingualism maintained despite no input from either home or community, some input at school, effect of six-month stay in Germany aged four. Positive effect of Saturday school.
Bindi	English, Gujarati	Kenya, UK	Two Gujarati parents. Fourth generation immigrant maintaining minority language, regrets not going to language school, couple changed language they spoke in front of the children, visiting Gujarat as an adult.

Name	Languages used as a child	As a child lived in	Particular issues arising
Camilla	Danish, English	UK	Two Danish parents, father Danish/English bilingual. Both parents spoke to her in Danish; after starting school she replied only in English, visited Denmark as a young adult, being shy and feeling different at school. Reaction to parental mistakes in majority language.
Charles	Dutch, French, Luxembourgian	Luxembourg, Holland	Initially 'one parent, one language' (OPOL) (Dutch/French) but his mother stopped speaking Dutch, maintained Dutch through school and later moved to Holland to study as an adult. Low impact of parental separation.
Christine	French, German	France	Initially OPOL (French/German) but her mother stopped speaking German to her age around seven, maintained German through holidays and through lessons at school.
Christopher	English, French	UK	OPOL plus French language school in London, effect of parents' divorce. Effect of changing school systems aged 16.
Claudia	English, German	Brazil, Namibia, Mozambique, Germany, Egypt	Two German-speaking parents. Mother decided to speak to the children in English. International schools, many moves.
Daniela	English, French, Italian	Italy, Switzerland, UK	Italian father, English mother, French at boarding school. Effect of parents' divorce. Learning a language at boarding school. Partially losing a language and resurrecting it.

Name	Languages used as a child	As a child lived in	Particular issues arising
Emilio	English, Spanish	Argentina	Father died when he was three, Spanish speaking mother. Learning English solely through school. Never exposed to English outside school until 18 years of age (except songs, films etc.)
Fatima	Arabic, English, French	Morocco, UK	Both parents speak Arabic. Bilingual education in Morocco, moved to UK aged 10, difficult transition in school, family with no common comfortably shared language.
Helen	Dutch, English	Holland	OPOL. Dutch mother, English father. Reluctant to speak English to her English father.
Ingrid	English, Swedish	Mexico, Sweden, USA (briefly)	Initially OPOL (American mother, Swedish father) but her father died when she was 11. Resisted responding to her mother in English until she was adult. Positive language classes at school, some other aspects of school negative.
Isabelle	English, French, Polish	Canada, France, USA	Learning a language from grandparents. OPOL English/Polish father spoke English, French mother. Effect of parents' divorce. Moves between countries affecting schooling. Retaining language through use between siblings only.
Josune	Basque, Spanish	Spain	Two Basque parents. Basque community with some Spanish. Strict rules within family regarding language use. Tension between children and parents on this point. Switch in language of education at university level – mainly unproblematic.

Name	Languages used as a child	As a child lived in	Particular issues arising
Kwesi	English, Fante, Twi	Ghana	Living in an international community, attending international school. Being viewed as an international without having international parentage or ever having travelled anywhere.
Marion	English, Welsh	UK	Living in extended family. Two bilingual English/Welsh parents. Tension within the family linked to language choices. Bilingualism interfering with progress at school, racism and teasing linked to language/nationality, a move of schools and country resolving problems aged 10.
Markus	English, German	USA, Germany	Mother English, father German. Extreme flexibility, switching mid-sentence, positive about language lessons at school, moving as an adult.
Matilde	French, Italian	Italy, Democratic Republic of Congo	Two Italian parents, aid workers lived in Africa. Moved age six, learned French, moved back to Italy and then again to Africa aged 11 and attended school in French, which she spoke but had never read or written. Feeling out of place after moving back to Italy aged 15.
Mohamed	Bengali/Sylheti, English	UK	Two Bengali parents, large family. Children's reluctance to speak Bengali is overcome by family. Racism at school and in the community, negative experiences at a language school. Very positive about being bilingual despite the above.

Name	Languages used as a child	As a child lived in	Particular issues arising
Mumtaz	English, Urdu	Pakistan, UK	Two Urdu speaking parents. Arrived in the UK aged seven and somewhat difficult transition in schooling, fell behind and hard to catch up. Family with no common language.
Pari	English, Gujarati	UK	Two Gujarati parents. Maintaining a language so as to be able to communicate with parents, family and community. Different behaviours with different languages. Not learning to read and write but not minding this.
Parvati	English, Hindi	UK	Two bilingual parents but one parent not totally supportive of minority language. Child carers supporting minority language. One language used more for discipline. Behaving differently depending on which language is being spoken. Feeling different at school, experiencing some racism.
Pedro	English, Spanish	USA	Two bilingual parents. Living in a community that routinely mixes languages. Living in a community segregated by language. Discrimination, low status language.
Rose	Cantonese, English, Hokkien, Mandarin	Singapore	National language policy – multilingualism through education policy, low impact of parental separation, her mother changed the language that she spoke to her as a child.
Saad	Arabic, Kurdish	Iraq, Kurdistan	Two Kurdish parents, father bilingual. Very consistent rules about language use at home. Speaking a language in a tense political context. Learning to read and write a language as an adult. Help with homework.

Name	Languages used as a child	As a child lived in	Particular issues arising
Saadia	English, Punjabi, Urdu	UK	Two Urdu speaking parents. Child choosing to change language spoken aged around 11. Regrets about not attending language school for longer. Positively wanting to be different linked to choice of language spoken.
Sabina	English, Urdu	UK	Child of two Urdu speaking parents, her mother died when she was nine, spoke mainly English for several years after this until her father remarried someone who only spoke Urdu. Learnt to read and write as an adult and regrets not learning as a child.
Sarah	English, German	Cameroon, Mauritius, Switzerland, UK	OPOL family, influence of school on OPOL at home. Humour within the family. Language and relationships.
Shadi	English, Farsi, French, Swedish	Iran, France, England, Sweden	Two Farsi speaking parents. Quadrilingual. Moved to Sweden aged 12 but learnt Swedish and education was not disrupted. Complex relationship to 'home country' – Iran.
Snjezana	Croatian, Esperanto, Italian	Croatia	Two (monolingual) Croatian parents. Taught Esperanto solely by her elder sister (despite parental discouragement), learnt Italian solely through attending Italian school, negative experiences at school, compartmentalised languages.
Sophie	French, Occitan Spanish	France	Two bilingual parents, extended family, additional Spanish speaking grandfather. Learning a language that is highly marginalised, learning from a grandparent, feeling different, not maintaining active use of one childhood language as an adult.

Name	Languages used as a child	As a child lived in	Particular issues arising
Susanne	English, German	Germany, UK	Two German parents, community and school English. Positive about Saturday school.
Sylvia	English, French	France	Two English parents, French from community and school. Very consistent English only at home rule, not fitting in, being different, finding peers at international school.
Tom	Croatian, English	Croatia, Australia	Two Croatian parents. Moved aged 11 with no English, found school difficult but managed. Became interested in Croatia and speaking Croatian again as an adult.
Velji	English, Gujarati, Swahili	Kenya	Two Gujarati parents. Learning one language through the community solely, learning another language through school. Third generation immigrant families retaining language. Learning to read and write a language as an adult.
Vera C	English, French	France	Childhood pre-Second World War. Having a strong accent.
Vera W	Cantonese, English	UK	Two Cantonese-speaking parents, school and community English. Strict rules about language used at home, speaking English to toys and siblings, racism at school, visiting China as an adult.
Zwelibanzi	English, Zulu	Zimbabwe	OPOL. Father decided to speak English to him at home and not Zulu for education/career reasons. English seen as a high-status language.

PART 1

Different Types of Family and Issues that Only Affect Some Kinds of Family

1 Issues for Families Speaking More than One Language at Home

2 Issues for Families Using One Language at Home, Another in the Community and at School

3 Interviewees who are Bilingual Solely through Attending School in Another Language

4 Interviewees who Learnt Languages Solely from the Community

5 Changes as a Result of Divorce or Separation

6 Changes as a Result of the Death of One Parent

7 Changes as a Result of Advice Given to Parents

8 Changes as a Result of Interviewees' Choices or Decisions

This section discusses the experiences of four main different kinds of multilingual settings that children grow up in and the factors and facets of life that affect only or primarily that type of family. I then discuss some of the families that experienced changes in their multilingual setting during their childhoods due to divorce or bereavement and then some changes due to the children's own choices.

The first group is composed of all the mixed-language families where each parent speaks a different language to the children. Here there are often decisions to be made about who speaks what language to the child(ren) and what language(s) the adults speak to each other. The second main group includes the families who speak one language at home and another at school and in the community. Many of these have moved – whether internationally or within a country. I discuss the different experiences of children who themselves remember moving as against those who were the children or grandchildren of migrants. I discuss what interviewees said about whether their parents could speak the majority language fluently or not. The third group is made up of the interviewees who learnt a language solely through attending a school that used a language other than the one they spoke at home as the main language medium to teach all or most subjects. These interviewees have learnt a language in isolation and have used it in quite limited settings and for limited purposes, and they may feel that they have some gaps in their vocabulary. Unless they continue to get input in the language after they leave the school, they will usually lose it. The fourth main group is those interviewees who learnt a language solely through their interactions with the community. It is interesting to discover that some children did learn a language quite quickly from what must have been quite limited input, although others in the same setting did not do so as they were not motivated to interact with the community as much.

I then share some accounts of how significant changes took place during some interviewees' childhoods as a result of divorce, bereavement, and as a result of advice given to parents. Finally in this section, I recount some remarkable instances of how children were active in making very positive and, in some cases, conscious choices about the languages that they spoke.

1 Issues for Families Speaking More than One Language at Home

Some issues are particularly relevant in mixed-language relationships, where the mother and father have different mother tongues. This may mean that at the outset of the relationship, or when children are born, parents have some choices to make about which language to speak between themselves and to the child(ren). This is even more the case if one or both parents are bilingual. So this chapter is for those who want to know more about how families have made these choices, how children remember them or what they were told about them and their impact as the children grew up. Interviewees discussed choices about what languages parents used to speak to the children, including where parents who were themselves bilingual made choices, where parents decided to speak a language other than a mother tongue to the children and what languages parents spoke between themselves. We also cover some examples where grandparents and other relatives were important in bringing another language to children.

Mixed Language Relationships – Languages Parents Used to Speak to the Children

It might seem automatic for those in a mixed-language relationship for each parent to speak their own first language to the children, and in most interviewees' families this was the case to the extent that it was almost taken for granted, and so many interviewees did not comment on this or raise it as an issue. Some families remember making decisions, or there was some doubt or discussion on this point. Where one or other parent decided not to speak their first, most fluent, or strongest language to the children, there was more awareness and usually some justification for the decision that was shared with the children later.

Armelle was the child of a Spanish-speaking mother from Argentina and a French father. Her mother who was then living in France sought advice about what language she should speak to her children: *'My mother told me that she went to a paediatrician [in France in the 1970s] when we were very young and she asked whether she could still speak Spanish to her children. He told her that she **should** speak Spanish to her children because she would be able to communicate her feelings better in her own language'*. Armelle's mother followed this advice (very consistently despite the fact that her children did not always reply to her in Spanish, and despite some adverse comments from other family members – see p.99). (Please note that not all doctors are as well informed about bilingualism as this one was. In fact, medical training does not cover this subject so if you want advice seek out a specialist in bilingualism.)

Helen was the child of an English father and a Dutch mother who had met and were living in Holland. When Helen was born, her father wanted her mother to speak English to her instead of Dutch. Dutch was Helen's mother's first language and she was not very fluent in English. Helen's mother found speaking English very difficult, and felt that it was artificial and preferred to speak in Dutch to her children. *'My father did feel a bit let down about this as though she didn't try hard enough, but she didn't feel natural'.* This seems to have been an unsuccessful attempt to achieve a more equal balance of English and Dutch within this family living in Holland. Although some individuals seem to have succeeded in speaking a language that was not their first language to their children (see Claudia, p.22), others find this very difficult (see also Sylvia, p.188).

Is a Mother's Influence Greater Than a Father's?

In our group, parents quite often wonder if it makes a difference whether a language is spoken to the children by a father or a mother – this concern often arises where fathers will be spending less time with young children. In our sample, this did not seem to be a significant factor. Where families did use a 'one person, one language' system, interviewees had as children learnt languages primarily from both mothers and fathers. This was the case even where schooling and the community were both in the mother's language and thus, together with the fact that the mother was spending more time with the children, this meant that quite a high proportion of a young child's input was in one language. So Helen's only input in English was from her father and from holidays in the UK – her mother spoke Dutch and the language used in the school and community was also Dutch. However, Helen speaks fluent English. Parvati's mother spoke a mixture of Hindi and English to her. Her father spoke only English to his children. Parvati's schooling was in English and she was raised in the UK, with occasional holidays in India. Nevertheless, she speaks fluent Hindi. Those interviewees who resisted speaking a parent's preferred language did so whether this was their mother's language (e.g. Ingrid, raised by an English-speaking mother and Swedish father in Sweden) or their father's (e.g. Helen. For more on this, see Chapter 11 on resistance).

One Bilingual Parent – Which Language?

In mixed-language families, where one or other parent is bilingual, there are three potential languages that can be spoken to the child(ren). In these families, it was more common for children to be aware of decisions or discussions about who spoke what language to the children. Several families who had the option seem to have decided not to raise their children trilingually. This was despite the fact that these families all included a successful bilingual adult, and so should not necessarily have been influenced by myths about children becoming confused by hearing several languages. Isabelle's Polish-Canadian father elected to speak English to his children. As he was married to a French woman this meant that the children still learnt two languages. In fact, Isabelle's (monolingual French) mother was keener on the children being raised bilingually than her already bilingual father was. Isabelle remembers that her mother argued for Isabelle to attend a bilingual French-English school: *'She was quite into languages herself ... she saw the value of it. It was because of her that we had the bilingual upbringing that we had. My father was much less fussed about it. He was like "they should integrate"'.*

Adeyinka's parents and Helen's mother both decided not to speak their first languages, which were local dialects to their children. In Adeyinka's case, he grew up speaking Yoruba at home in Nigeria but attended an English-medium school. Both his parents spoke different dialects of Yoruba, but they both spoke mainly standard Yoruba to their children, meaning that the children only learnt standard Yoruba and neither of their parents' dialects. In Helen's Dutch-English family, her mother was a bilingual Dutch and Frisian speaker where the family agreed that it might be too confusing to try to bring the children up speaking three languages and Frisian was not spoken at home, although Helen learnt at least some Frisian from her Dutch grandmother who she saw regularly.

When faced with a bilingual parent who has a choice between two languages, there seem to be two opposite ways that a family can go: either to opt for a more widely-spoken language, often a language widely perceived as having a higher status or being seen as more useful, or to opt for a dialect or less widely-spoken language. Thus standard forms can be preferred over dialects, national languages over local ones and, as mentioned above, in Isabelle's family in Canada, English was preferred over Polish. However, some families do take the other tack, and choose to speak either a dialect or a less widely-spoken language to their children in preference to a more internationally used language. So Josune has decided to speak Basque and not Spanish to her children (who are also learning English and Czech), and Saad has decided to speak Kurdish and not Arabic to his children. Josune specifically explains her decision in terms of the children having little chance of learning Basque in later life if they did not learn it from her, whereas they would have a much better chance of learning Spanish from other sources. In several cases where the family decided to opt for a more widely-spoken language, either the child or the parent regretted this decision later. So, for example, Adeyinka wished that both his parents had spoken the same dialect so that he could have learnt that and become trilingual, and Helen's mother has said that she regrets not raising Helen to also speak more Frisian.

In multilingual Luxembourg, Charles's bilingual French/Luxembourgian-speaking father chose to speak French to his children, whilst his bilingual Dutch-French mother started out speaking to them in Dutch. The children also heard Luxembourgian in the community at large. Charles thinks his mother's decision to speak Dutch to her children was a reaction to her own childhood *'because when she was growing up... She grew up in Holland and her mother wanted them to speak French rather than Dutch so her and her sister were speaking in Dutch and her mother wanted them to speak French. In Holland, back in those days, [French] was a sign of high society. She wanted us to know Dutch, because she really liked Dutch language and she was very proud of it'.* In fact, as the children grew older Charles's mother struggled to stick to her initial decision and gradually switched to speaking more and more French.

Two Bilingual Parents – What Mix of Languages?

Some interviewees grew up in families where both parents had been bilingual since childhood; a Spanish-speaking family in Texas, a family speaking Occitan and French in south-western France, a Welsh family in London and Wales, and a family speaking Hindi and English in the UK. In these families there is inherently more choice and more flexibility in both the languages used between adults and in who speaks what language to the children. In two of these four examples, there was considerable use of both languages by both parents as well as by the children, including some switching or mixing of languages.

Pedro was born and brought up in a small town in Texas, in the United States of America. Most people in the area spoke Spanish at home. In Pedro's family, his parents primarily spoke to the children in Spanish. His father was more consistent in speaking Spanish; he did not mix English and Spanish, whereas Pedro's mother would mix the two languages freely: *'With my Dad, whatever language he spoke to you, you responded in that language ... if he spoke to you in English, you responded in English, if he spoke in Spanish, you responded in Spanish. With my Mum if she spoke to you in Spanish, it was OK if you replied in English'.*

His father would query if the children spoke 'Spanglish' or a mixture of Spanish and English to him. *'One thing we didn't do was speak Spanglish to him. He didn't tolerate that. If you spoke Spanglish to him, he would let you know. He would say "Speak English, or speak Spanish, don't mix the languages"'.*

Pedro says that his father's choice of language did not follow a particular pattern but: *'It depended on what mode his mind was on ...'.* He gives the example of when his father had been watching TV (which at that time was only in English) he would be 'in English mode' and would probably speak in English.

Another example of parents switching or mixing languages concerns Sophie, who was born and brought up in south-west France, not far from Bordeaux. She grew up in an extended family where her parents, and initially four grandparents and an 'adopted grandfather', all lived in adjoining buildings close together. The whole family ate lunch and dinner together every day and there was a close connection between them all. The whole of her family spoke both French and Occitan. Occitan has some similarities in vocabulary and grammar to Spanish, Italian and Portuguese. Linguists regard it as a distinct language, but in France it is commonly seen either as a dialect or a degraded version of French. When she was a child, Sophie's grandparents and parents would speak to her in both French and Occitan at home. She thinks that generally one of her grandparents would initiate a conversation in Occitan and her father would reply in either French or Occitan, while her mother would reply more often in French. Thus she heard both French and Occitan at home, whether spoken directly to her or in conversations amongst the adults. Sophie herself mostly responded in French, however, and only occasionally spoke Occitan herself.

Marion

In contrast, although Marion's family could all speak and understand both Welsh and English, there were very clear and fixed patterns within the family about who spoke what language to whom. Marion grew up in South London where she was living with her Welsh family until the age of nine. She lived in a house that was split into two flats. Marion, her parents and her older sister lived on the top floor, and her grandparents (from her mother's side) lived on the bottom floor. She spoke English with her mother, sister and grandfather, and Welsh with her father and grandmother. There were distinct ways of using language in the house that cut across the three generations. Her grandmother spoke fluent Welsh (from South Wales), but her grandfather (from the border) spoke some Welsh, but not fluently. *'He mocked my grandmother at speaking Welsh ... it being old fashioned. You wouldn't get ahead if you spoke Welsh'.*

In contrast, Marion's father was very pro-Welsh: *'Although he worked for the [British] government at the time [my father] was still very Welsh, very pro-Wales, a supporter of Welsh nationalism and his family is from North Wales, and North Wales is the bastion of the Welsh language. My mother, very much sided with her pro-English father, spoke English all the time, although she could understand Welsh completely and she read fluently, but she refused to use the language; almost consistently through the whole of the time that I knew her. My sister was very much like my mother and has very little Welsh ...'.*

Marion's father spoke Welsh to his mother-in-law and English to his wife. Marion's father's mother in Wales spoke no English: *'All her grandchildren had to speak some Welsh'.*

'When I was growing up, my father was committed to make me Welsh speaking and I spent a lot of time being looked after by my grandmother, because my mother went back to work. And my father also took a lot of responsibility for me and we did everything in Welsh. I must have grown up with a kind of mix of English and Welsh until the age of five. When I got to school in London, where nobody spoke Welsh, I was more comfortable with Welsh'. Marion's early education in English was not straightforward (this is described on p.111).

Marion clearly feels that the disputed language division in her family was not helpful. This contributed to her decision not to raise her own children fully bilingually: *'I don't want to build up an environment in the way that I grew up where it really divided the family into two. I was very much my father's daughter, and my sister was very much my mother's daughter. It [language] really split the family down the middle'.* Marion's advice to other families is to avoid such a split occurring: *'It's very important the child is aware that the family is not divided and that both parents are seen to invest in the two, three languages, so that even if one of them doesn't speak it they are clearly happy with the other one speaking it'.*

The final case involves Parvati, whose Indian father had first learnt Hindi as a very young child, but increasingly switched to English after learning it at school and he spoke almost exclusively in English to his children. Parvati's parents were both Indian and moved to the UK in the 1960s as young adults. Both of her parents spoke Hindi and English (Parvati's mother also spoke Urdu and Punjabi). Parvati's mother had learnt English informally as a child. She had travelled to the UK for short periods during her childhood, and she had fluent colloquial but not academic English. Parvati's father had learnt English at school and attended a high-status English-medium university in India. Parvati's mother spoke to her husband in a mixture of Hindi and English and he replied almost always in English (unless he did not want white British people around to understand what he was saying). Both Parvati and her older sister were born in the UK. At home Parvati's mother spoke to her in a mixture of English and Hindi, but her father spoke exclusively English, and both girls spoke only English to him.

Parvati explains that her father: *'left India to seek a better life for himself and his family in an intellectual sense … he really wanted us to have educational opportunities. He was not a typical Indian man, a lot of Indian families have a Bollywood culture in the background, (i.e. they watch a lot of Bollywood films and some have the films and the TV series as a constant backdrop), we did have a bit of that but only through my mother and my aunts, but my father doesn't speak Hindi if he can avoid it'.* Later in the interview, Parvati also said: *'My father has this snobbery, which I think we initially inherited, but soon discarded, about speaking Hindi being a bit low class …'.*

These families where both parents are themselves multilingual might seem to have advantages over others. However, although all of these interviewees did learn both languages, Sophie does not speak Occitan today although she still understands it. (She does speak four other languages fluently.) Neither Marion nor Pedro chose to raise their children speaking the minority language (Spanish and Welsh) and, of this group, Parvati was the interviewee who conveyed the most confidence and who seemed most comfortable speaking Hindi. It is not clear from our group that the system used within the family was in any way a determining factor. Families ranged from the very fluid 'everybody speaks everything', to those where there were clear and consistent divisions. However, it does seem to me to be almost certainly significant that three of these four situations involve heavily marginalised languages (Spanish in Texas, Welsh in London and Occitan in France). There are other examples in the book of interviewees raised speaking marginalised languages with no difficulty at all. However, where a language is marginalised it may be important that there is a political or cultural movement in support of that language – at least something that tells children that a language is something to be proud of. Neither Pedro nor Sophie's family engaged at all with the very limited movements that existed at that time in support of Spanish or Occitan. In Marion's case there was a well-established movement supporting Welsh, which her father was clearly part of. However, Marion's situation was complicated by the split within the family, which she clearly found difficult. Overall, this does suggest that the value placed on the language in the family and in the community is far more important than multilingual families commonly suppose.

What if One Parent Does not Understand the Conversations Between the Other Parent and the Children?

Some families attending our group have expressed concerns if, for example, the mother is speaking Urdu to the children but the father neither speaks nor understands

Urdu. Sometimes they worry about one parent being excluded from an important part of family life because of the other parent's choice of language. They also wonder about sending mixed messages to the children from the parents and confusion, or even the children being able to manipulate this in terms of discipline. Only one of our interviewees grew up in a family where one parent did not understand the language that the other parent used to speak to the children. This was Christopher, the son of a French mother and English father who grew up in London. The fact that his father, an osteopath, could not understand French was not an issue for this family. *'It did not bother him in the least ... He was English, but he liked the French people and he liked going to France, but he could never speak French'.*

As adults, some of our interviewees did refer to this factor as affecting their decisions about the language that they have chosen to speak to their children. See also Adeyinka (p.189) who says that the fact that his wife does not speak Yoruba has inhibited him from speaking Yoruba to his daughter.

In one case, the fact that at least some of the family conversations were taking place in a language that was not one parent's first language did sometimes affect family dynamics in more subtle ways. Sarah, who is a German-English bilingual whose mother speaks good but not native English, is aware that joking in English can make her mother feel left out at times. Sarah, her brother, and her father, who is a big joker, like cracking jokes in English. *'[My mother] is "funnier" in German, a lot funnier, in fact she is very, very funny in German, but she is not so good at it in English. She will perceive what's going on, and she will understand the delicacies of what's making it funny, but she wouldn't be able to add to it and that makes it very difficult for her sometimes ... sometimes depending on her mood, she can sit back, and she can just let it happen and enjoy it.... Sometimes she would come out with something in German. I can respond to her, my brother can a little bit, but my father can't as much...but it breaks the flow of it, a little bit. It is a little tricky. ... Watching my parents negotiate this multilingualism, there has been an interesting thing in terms of my decision... in relation to finding a partner. I'm really aware of how much of an impact it can actually have not to be able to share humour with your partner. They [my parents] share a lot of other things, but the humour part is not as good as it could be. I'm really aware of that'.*

Our interviews did not really shed light on the issue of one parent not understanding conversations between the other parent and the child(ren), but many families have developed a range of strategies to deal with this. In some families the second parent has actually been able to learn enough of the language to understand these important conversations, whereas in others important messages are simply repeated in the common language. Provided that the second parent is relaxed about and supportive of the use of the language that they do not understand, it seems that families can function perfectly well in this way.

Parents Who Chose not to Speak their First Language to their Children

There were two examples of this. I was particularly interested in them as they go against the most common advice to parents. I am very familiar from my discussions at

WFBG and my reading on this subject that most professionals will normally advise any bilingual family just setting out that they should: 'Speak your first/your most fluent language to your children'. I have mentioned above (p.16) the discussion within Helen's family about her speaking English and not her native Dutch to her children, and her attempts that were unsuccessful. Other interviewees referred to their own difficulties in speaking a particular language to their own children (see Sylvia, p.188). But there were two examples amongst our samples where a parent did decide to do this and was very successful (there is even an example of a sibling doing so, see Snjezana, p.26).

The most extreme example is that of Claudia who is a German-English bilingual. Unusually, Claudia was raised bilingually by two parents who were both mother tongue German speakers. Although both her parents spoke excellent English, they had only learnt this as adults. (Claudia's mother now teaches English and her use of the language is indistinguishable from that of a native English speaker.) Her mother had not learned any significant English before the age of 19 but loved the language and all things English, which led to her decision to raise her children bilingually in a language she had learnt as an adult. Combined with this was the fact that Claudia's father was a diplomat and her parents knew that she would need to attend international schools as they moved around the world, and that, in many postings, English would be the common language in the diplomatic community (for more on Claudia, see p.73).

The other example concerns Zwelibanzi, whose Zimbabwean father elected to speak to him in English – particularly after he was five years old. Zwelibanzi's father's first language was Zulu although he had also learnt to speak fluent English at school and was a civil servant, and so spoke English daily at his work. Zwelibanzi thinks his parents encouraged him to speak English so he could succeed at school. *'It was prestigious to talk in English. … If you speak English it means you've got guaranteed work because it is an official language'.*

Of course it was important that, in both of these cases we encountered, the parents involved were very fluent in and had a very good knowledge of the language that they chose to speak to their children. Perhaps it is not a coincidence that in both cases the language selected was English, because of the perceived high prestige and usefulness of English as an international language.

Terms for Mummy, Daddy and Other Family Members

One interesting side issue that arises within the area of the choice of language spoken to the children is the terms used to refer to the parents and other relatives. If you remain speaking the same language consistently, it will mean that one person (e.g. the father) is referred to by different terms depending on who is speaking. Children will soon learn that 'Papa' and 'Daddy' mean the same thing (although my own daughter caused confusion at one stage by asserting 'I don't have a Daddy'. Clearly she did not consider her Papa the same thing). I feel that it may be useful symbolically for both parents to switch into the other's language for these terms. This will mean that each parent is consistently referred to by one term – the term in the language that they speak to the children. In Helen's case, her English father living in Holland was referred to as Papa, the Dutch term, and interestingly Helen says: *'I do now regret that I didn't call him "Daddy" but called him "Papa" – father in Dutch'.* Once made and established, these choices cannot be easily changed. They may seem very small and insignificant, but as these terms are amongst the first that children learn to both understand and say, and as they are then repeated daily many times over, they may have more significance than might at first appear, particularly in terms of their symbolism.

Many mixed language families have a 'Maman' and a 'Daddy', or a 'Mummy' and a 'Baba'. These terms are like names, and so can always be used no matter which language is being spoken. One interviewee, when describing telling her parents about her decision to speak German to her child, said, for example, *'I've told them that I'm speaking German to our son and that I want "Oma" and "Opa" to speak German to him'.* (Oma means grandma and opa means grandpa in German.)

Even within the nuclear family, this may not feel very natural initially and may need a conscious decision and a discussion, rather than simply allowing what seems most obvious to emerge. It may also be helpful if wider family members (e.g. grandparents and uncles and aunts) also follow this rule, which is even less likely to happen without a conscious decision and discussion – especially if the wider family do not speak the language in question.

Languages Used Between Parents

From conversations with WFBG members, I get the impression that parents in multilingual families tend to think most about the languages that they actually speak directly to children. This clearly *is* important, but this should not lead us to underestimate the influence of the language spoken by adults in conversations that the children hear but do not participate in. One reason that conversations between adults are almost equally important is that they are more complex and can be very varied compared to the conversations that take place between adults and children, which can be both quite simple and quite repetitive – particularly when children are still young. If only one language is chosen as the language used between the parents, and if this is also the majority language, it will inevitably mean that quite a high proportion of all the speech that a children hears is in that language. The choice of languages spoken between adults is also important symbolically, particularly in terms of the messages it conveys to children about the value of languages. Not all couples have a free choice on this issue. In some cases in our sample of interviewees, although their parents had learnt the language at school or as adults, they were both competent speakers or even fluent in both languages, but in other cases, neither had spoken the other's language well when they met. Where this was the case, often one parent still acquired a very good knowledge of the other's language over time, particularly if it was widely spoken where they lived.

The language used between the parents was normally established when they met and was often influenced by their relative language skills at that particular moment; so, in Sarah's case, when they were together as a family they spoke mostly in English because her mother's English was better than her father's German. I wondered if this might be determined by the language of the country they were in when they met or first lived together, but there were several examples of couples choosing the other language. There were no examples among our interviewees where the parents deliberately chose to speak one parent's weaker language in order to help that parent develop their knowledge and fluency in the language, although WFBG includes several families as members who have done so at the outset of a relationship, particularly where this language is the majority language where they are living. The relative strength of two parents' languages may change over time, but often the language of the relationship will become fixed and may be difficult to change even after the original reasons for the decision no longer apply. For example: Helen grew up in the Netherlands with a Dutch mother and an English father. Neither of her parents spoke the other's language well when they met. They spoke in English together and have continued to do so, although Helen's father has since learnt to speak excellent Dutch.

One interviewee commented on the choice of language between herself and her husband as adults, and noted that it was more important that they could both operate at an equal level than that they speak the languages that they individually knew best: *'It's a bit of a power game. We cannot have a satisfactory conversation in any other language, either I speak the language much better (e.g. English) or he can (e.g. German)'*. So some couples may pick a language that they both speak at the same level as part of an equal relationship.

As in this example, in most cases the parents settled on one language that they both used; however, in one case, the parents each used their own first language to address the other. Armelle's father always spoke to his wife in French and she only replied in Spanish – thus they had a truly bilingual relationship. Both parents can speak fluently in the other's language if necessary (i.e. to a monolingual speaker). There is a certain logic to this, and certainly it provides the children with input from adults speaking both languages in adult conversations, so it is perhaps surprising that this seems to be so rare.

What is clear is that couples establish a habitual language of communication amongst themselves. They build up considerable emotional memories in that language, and they may have shared jokes and phrases in that language. They then find it very difficult to switch at a later point, when it may make sense to do so for the sake of the children. There were more examples in our interviews of parents changing the language that they spoke to children than there were of parents changing the language used between the couple. For example, Markus's parents were both fluent in German and English (his mother was English and his father German). They would vary the amount of German and English that they spoke to their children to try to balance out changes in the external environment, as the family moved back and forwards several times between the United States and Germany. Despite this clear and deliberate flexibility with regard to the languages spoken to the children (described in more detail below, see p.73), Markus recalls that his parents spoke mainly English between themselves throughout these moves and language changes. We are also aware of several families who have tried to change the language spoken between the adults, but quickly fall back into established language habits. Some families have tried and succeeded so it is possible, if rare (see Bindi, p.190).

Your family may be the exception to this rule, but otherwise, you may have to be very determined and persistent if you want to change the language spoken between a couple, whether this is to provide a better language balance for the children or for other reasons.

Extended Families: Bilingualism as a Result of the Input of Other Relatives

Until now we have mainly been talking in terms of nuclear families, with one or two parents living with their children. Although both Sophie's and Marion's grandparents were important influences, they were speaking the same languages as their parents. But there were several other examples where grandparents and other relatives had an important role in introducing a totally different language to children.

Spanish from an Adopted Grandfather (with Additional Input) and Italian from Grandparents

Sophie, the Occitan/French speaker, also learnt Spanish as a child. She lived in south-western France near Bordeaux with her father, mother and four grandparents. Also living with them was a Spanish 'adopted grandfather', a refugee who had fled from Franco's regime to live in France and was taken in by Sophie's family, and who had lived with them ever since. His mother tongue was Spanish, but he also spoke fluent French and Occitan. Sophie's adopted grandfather had always spoken some Spanish to her as a young child – they would talk to together about what they were doing or things in the environment, and he would explain things to her in both Spanish and French. This may well not have been enough for Sophie to establish and maintain Spanish, but it certainly gave her major advantages when she started studying it at school aged 10. She went to this adopted grandfather and asked him to speak Spanish to her more systematically, and he also helped her with her Spanish homework. Sophie loved her Spanish lessons at school. She was very good at the language and would sometimes give the teacher input or suggest words that were not actually intended to be covered in the lesson (which she had previously learned from her grandfather). Fortunately, the teacher responded to this in a good-humoured way and did not discourage her. The level of Spanish that she had gained by speaking to her grandfather was not so great, though, that she was bored by the lessons or felt that she was learning nothing. She also feels that her knowledge of Occitan, which shares some links with Spanish, Portuguese and Italian, may have helped her to learn Spanish. Subsequently, Sophie lived in Spain for a year when she was 17 and attended school there. Although the parents in her host family could speak French, and would occasionally use a French word to help Sophie out, she spoke and heard almost exclusively Spanish, and by the end of the year she was totally fluent.

An example of an interviewee gaining some command of a language from grandparents up to the age of six is Isabelle, who was the daughter of a French mother and Polish-Canadian father. Her paternal grandparents did speak English, but they were more comfortable speaking Polish. Isabelle remembers spending a lot of time with them – cooking with her grandma or running out to greet her grandpa when he got back from work. Isabelle could interact competently with them (at the level of a six-year-old) in Polish. Through her grandparents, Isabelle would meet other Polish speakers in the community, but not many children her own age. Then, when Isabelle was six, the family (by then including her younger brother) moved to Atlanta and the children no longer had the Polish input from their grandparents. In later years, Isabelle visited her grandparents once in Quebec City and they visited her once in Atlanta, but she did not have very much contact with her grandparents after she left the United States when she was nine. Later, whilst she was at university in the United States, she managed to get onto a Polish course, although she needed to do two language courses to get her Polish to the level whereby she could get onto the programme to study Polish culture in Polish. Eventually she was able to go to Poland for a term to study, and she now speaks very competent Polish.

Esperanto from a Mainly Croatian-Speaking Older Sister

Linked to the above group, but uniquely in this book, Snjezana was born to two monolingual Croatian speakers and lived all of her childhood in Croatia. In Snjezana's case the second language input came from her eldest sister, who is 12 years older than her. This sister had begun learning Esperanto, was doing a correspondence course and needed someone to practise speaking the language with, and decided to teach her baby sister. She spoke Esperanto to Snjezana from when Snjezana was a small baby. *'She [Snjezana's sister] claims that I started speaking Croatian and Esperanto at the same time'.*

Snjezana's sister did not exclusively speak Esperanto though, as Snjezana's mother and father (who did not speak the language) were resistant to this scheme and, in fact, tried unsuccessfully to ban it. Until she was 14, almost all of Snjezana's Esperanto input was from conversations with her eldest sister. At times, as well as in everyday conversations, this would be more like formal teaching when they would talk about a particular subject. Despite this unusual style and limited level of input, Snjezana spoke Esperanto well, possibly because: *'I am close to this sister. We spent quite a lot of time together'.*

At some point, Snjezana does not remember exactly when, the Esperanto conversations with her sister stopped and she no longer spoke Esperanto. She speculates that this may have been because she had more homework and needed to concentrate more on her studies, or, alternatively, she now wonders whether they finally gave in to the pressure from her parents. However, when she was 14 (and her sister 26), they had the opportunity to go to an annual Esperanto event abroad. This was a great opportunity for Snjezana and her sister to travel and see new places, which they very much appreciated. *'The first time we went to Poland [to an Esperanto event]; it took me a while to get back into the swing of [speaking Esperanto]'*.

So from this point on, Snjezana and her sister started speaking Esperanto together again. Finally, when she was 23, Snjezana met her husband at an Esperanto event. He is Hungarian and Esperanto is their common language. *'I never formally learnt Esperanto. I can read and write when necessary, but I have never had a chance to use it professionally, I consider it a household language'*.

Conclusion

There may well be more ways of arranging the languages spoken within the family than most people in multilingual families are aware of. See page 212 for some ideas on assessing how much input your child(ren) are getting or will get in each language.

- Consider what language(s) each parent will speak to the child. If at all possible, start as you mean to go on. There are many different successful strategies. Find something that gives the children a reasonable balance but feels OK to you. (It is harder to sustain something that does not feel natural to you but remember that, provided that the children are introduced to it at birth or in their first few months, it will feel totally natural and 'just the way things are' to them) (see also Chapter 30).
- Consider what language the parents will speak to each other; do not underestimate the impact on children of hearing adult speech.
- If you both understand both languages, do not discount the possibility that each parent could speak their own language to each other – a truly bilingual relationship.
- It is a big and difficult decision to speak a language that is not your first language or mother tongue to your child(ren). It is certainly true that you need to speak a language very well to speak it as the main language to your children (and you need to bear in mind that it is the breadth of idioms and expressions, nursery rhymes, jokes and sayings that children's language thrives on – not the basic day-to-day conversations about meals, baths and daily life). But our interviewees showed that several families did choose to do this – some tried but said that it felt too unnatural, while others were highly successful. Again, remember that whatever a child has grown up with will feel natural to him or her (there is a whole website devoted to families in this situation, see http://babybilingual.blogspot.com/2010/01/deux.html).
- If you do want to change the language one of the adults speaks to the child or to other adults, do not underestimate the difficulty of doing so; language habits are as difficult to change once established, as with any other habit – and possibly more difficult (see also Chapter 30).

- We would advise that you do not change your language pattern after your child has reached three months, and until your child has reached the stage of being aware of different languages so, for example, until your child makes statements like 'grandma speaks English, aunty speaks Urdu'.
- Think about terms in your language for people (e.g. words for mummy, daddy, grandma). See if you can enlist everyone's help to use the same terms for key people.
- Do not seek advice about bilingualism from anyone who is not a specialist in bilingualism. If you are offered unsolicited advice from those who do not have a specialism in bilingualism, treat it with caution.
- Be aware that if you are yourself bilingual and you choose not to speak a lesser-used language to your children, although they will value the language that they have, they may also regret not learning a dialect, local language or Creole. In many situations where parents opt for a lesser-used language, the child(ren) will nonetheless learn a major international language (opt for Kurdish, and the children will learn Arabic anyway, opt for Basque and the children will learn Spanish anyway) whereas the reverse is not true. On the other hand, the level of resources available and the prestige linked to major international languages makes sustaining a child's use of a language easier and more likely to succeed. Probably one of the most important factors in this whole project is your emotional commitment to the minority language(s) you want your children to speak, so, regardless of the above, my advice to you would be to select the language you feel you have the strongest feelings for.
- Whatever you decide to do, make sure that it is a joint project. If one parent speaks the majority language and one a minority language, the support of the majority language-speaking parent is very important. In particular, it is essential that he or she does not disparage or undermine the minority language or culture in any way. It is also very important that you do not air disagreements or doubts about the decisions you have taken about the languages you are each speaking in front of the children. Children will be quick to pick up on divisions, and differences of opinion between parents. Even much subtler, but still disparaging, comments were noted by interviewees. We were struck by the fact that several interviewees remembered word for word disparaging or negative comments about one or other language decades later. This was the case even though the comments were usually addressed to the other parent or another adult – not to the child themselves.
- If one parent does not understand the minority language you can encourage them to gain a passive knowledge of it as the child learns. This is easier than it might sound, as the vocabulary used to and by very young children is very simple and quite limited. If a partner learns in this way from the birth of a child, even when the children are school age, a monolingual partner may well be able to understand the gist of many significant conversations about disciplinary issues ('No more biscuits until after tea! Do you want an apple?') in another language.
- If you will be raising your children to speak a language that is not recognised or high status in the community where you live, think carefully about how you can bolster

support for that language by mixing with other families who speak it, or by going out of your way to convey to your children how much you value the language.

- Do not underestimate the influence of grandparents and other relatives if they live near to you or with you in providing support for a language.
- Finally, remember that all our interviewees speaking more than one language at home were pleased that they had been raised multilingually. All were glad to be able to speak more than one language. No one remembered being confused or ever having wished that they were not bilingual.

2 Issues for Families Using One Language at Home, Another in the Community and at School

There is another set of issues that are relevant for families who speak one language at home and another in the community. In all the cases in our sample, this was due to the fact that they or their parents or grandparents had migrated to a new country. Just over 20 of our interviewees received input in a second and/or third language that was not spoken at home from the community. In this group, it was clear that the interviewees' experiences depended a lot on how old they were when they moved. There are two groups – those who remember life in a previous country and the process of adjusting to life in a new setting, and those who do not. Some experiences stem from the fact that their parents did not speak the language of their new country perfectly or at all well. So some recall hearing their parents speak with an accent or making mistakes in the majority language, and some interviewees helped as interpreters or to complete forms or similar tasks in that language – with a strikingly wide range of responses and reactions from the children involved. Some interviewees felt that they did not gain a full understanding of the country their family had moved to or felt that they did not fully belong (see also Chapter 22).

Some interviewees were born in the country that they grew up in (primarily the UK, but also Australia and Kenya), and this group was more likely to speak Asian languages at home – Cantonese, Gujarati and Urdu – with also some European languages – Danish, German and Greek. Twice as many interviewees had moved as children with their families. Some had moved to Europe to take up opportunities for work (mainly from Africa and Asia – e.g. Morocco, Kenya, Bangladesh or Pakistan to the UK). Some had migrated within Europe to take up work opportunities (e.g. France to Italy, Germany to the UK, and the UK to France). Some had fled their country of origin due to political upheavals as refugees (e.g. Iran to Europe, Cyprus to the UK). There was also one Italian interviewee within this group whose father who was a medical doctor worked for a development agency that led the family to spend around seven years in what was then Zaire (now the Democratic Republic of Congo).

Many of those migrating to Europe as refugees or economic migrants were themselves the elite in their home countries with high-levels of education (e.g. Shadi's Iranian father who had a PhD) and who had worked as professionals before they moved (e.g. Mohammed's father had been a schoolteacher in Bangladesh). At the other end of the spectrum, the sample did include a number of children of poorer and less well-educated migrants.

Overall there is a contrast in our group of interviewees between those moving into as opposed to away from Europe and North America. Most of the migrants into Europe were much more likely to only move once. Most saw it as a permanent move, did not envisage returning home to live and in most cases their parents put more emphasis on children integrating fully into the culture of the new country. For example, Saadia's parents felt that it was important that their children spoke very good English to do well in life in England: *'We were instilled with the sense that English is very important and that to do well you had to be well spoken'*.

Families moving within Europe/North America or from Europe/North America to the South were more likely to move several times and to see their stay in a particular country as purely linked to a particular career move or assignment and as quite temporary. These interviewees often attended international schools and their home language was generally a relatively high status language. These families did not place the same emphasis on integration within the new country.

The Age Interviewees Moved

For those that moved with their families, one important factor was the age at which they moved. This ranged from 13 months to 12 years old. We did not interview anyone who had moved away from their home country when they were already over 12 years old (although we were told about interviewees' sisters and brothers who had). In the case of interviewees who moved when they were under the age of four, they had usually had a very limited interaction with the community in the country of origin, and often no memories of living there. Whilst several interviewees picked up some of a local language at this age, unless it was also one of their parent's languages, they quickly lost it when they moved.

In discussing the ages interviewees moved between language environments, Astrid is an interesting case. She was born in Australia. Her parents had both come to Australia from Germany when they were teenagers, both were bilingual German-English speakers and they decided to speak English when they got married and had children because they wanted to integrate into the community. When Astrid was four the family spent six months in Germany and this seems to have made a big impression on her. *'My mum says I didn't speak any English when I came back to Australia! I think it gave me the grounding. I think German stayed with me. I always wanted to speak it. I think I learned so much in those six months. When I picked it up again when I started German Saturday school and later at the university I found it quite easy, it just came naturally to me whereas with my sister [who is several years younger and so missed out on this experience] it was quite different'*. Astrid was the youngest child who retained some of the language she had spoken before her move – all the more impressive as she was only in Germany for six months. (Of course in most other cases, the parents continued to speak the language concerned to the children after the move.)

The interviewees who moved after they were around five or six years old had usually started school in their home country and have clear memories of living there. These interviewees were making a transition between two languages and cultures, compared to the interviewees who moved younger who were negotiating a mainstream and a home language which was all that they had ever really known. The interviewees who moved later were clearly aware of the transition and this sometimes made things more difficult for them. After his move from Croatia to Australia aged 11, Tom, for example, remembers that he felt homesick and missed his friends from Croatia. More than two decades later, Tom went back to Croatia for the first time and was looking for a friend from his school days. *'That was the only conflict I had. I still missed my roots. My younger brother and sister never felt that way. They assimilated much better in all ways than I did'.*

Another child who moved relatively late was Fatima. Her father left Morocco to take up a catering contact in the UK in the 1960s. Initially he went on his own and just visited the family regularly, but in 1973, when Fatima was seven, he arranged for Fatima's mother to join him. It was difficult to bring children to the UK, so, at first, all the children stayed in Morocco – divided between the two sets of grandparents. A year later Fatima's eldest brother came to join their parents, and in 1976, when Fatima was 10, the rest of the children were able to come to the UK. Fatima's eldest brother was 18 when he came to the UK, and her youngest brother was born here. The other children spanned this gap. The age that they made this move affected how they reacted and how they got on. Fatima was 10, but her younger sister was five when they came to the UK: *'It was harder for her ... I remember her being bullied in school. It was quite traumatic for her. Having not had her parents there, then coming here and being thrown into this environment'.* Fatima's siblings also show a range of fluency in Arabic and English according to the age that they moved. So her eldest brother does speak and understand English but is much more confident speaking Arabic, while her youngest brother is much more fluent in English than Arabic. The middle children are much more balanced bilinguals. Fatima also told us that she felt that her sister's transition in terms of education was easier than her own (see p.113).

Armelle and Claudia are both interesting because they moved country without changing the language of their education, and this confirms the expectation that this would have much less impact on them. (However, for a contrasting experience, see Aimee's account on p.119.) As a young child, Armelle had already moved three times, from Spain where she was born, to Paris, and then to Argentina. When she was seven, French and Spanish-speaking Armelle moved from Argentina (where she attended an international French/bilingual school) to Italy (where she attended the international French school). Armelle did not feel that this move was disruptive or problematic. Claudia's German and English-speaking diplomatic family moved around a lot – including moves between Mozambique and Namibia – but as she attended an English language school in both countries, these moves were much less notable than the next one, which was back to Germany where Claudia attended German school – changing both the language medium and an international school for an ordinary German school. (This seemed a big change to her despite the fact that Claudia spoke both German and English at home and was fluent in both languages. See also page 116).

One interviewee, Matilde, moved when she was 15 back to Italy from Zaire (where her father who was a doctor had been working for an aid organisation), which she found difficult, but mainly for cultural reasons. She had already lived in Italy as a much younger child and her family had consistently spoken Italian at home. Although her family mainly spoke Italian, they did mix French and Swahili words into sentences. When Matilde got back to Italy this was a problem as she found it difficult to say a whole sentence without using French or Swahili words and her friends noticed this. But for Matilde the transition was mainly about culture and identity: *'We were always the weird family. People back in Italy found it strange that my family had lived in Africa. ... It's difficult when you're fifteen. That was the most difficult part. Teenagers have their rules, and I had been used to society in Goma [in Zaire]'.* And she added later in the interview that, *'... when I first came back to Italy from Goma, despite the fact that I had wanted to come back to Italy, I felt that I belonged in Goma, I was fifteen, most of my memories until then had been in Africa and I didn't feel like I belonged in Italy'.*

Interviewees who moved when they were already at school also involved moves between education systems, but this is a big topic and is dealt with in Chapter 14.

Could Migrant Parents Speak the Majority Language in the New Country?

One factor that affected the experiences of this group was the degree to which the parents were able to function in the majority language. This varied from parents who were completely fluent to those who were beginners, and everything in between. There was also a difference in that some interviewees belonged to families with at least one competent or fluent speaker, and some interviewees had two parents who did not speak the majority language well.

Mohammed's schoolteacher father came from Bangladesh to live in the UK. Mohammed was aware that his father spoke English well – he would speak English in front of his children at parents' evenings and similar interactions with the school. He also wrote very accurately and formally in English, and would write any notes needed for school.

In many other cases, although interviewees' parents had good levels of a language that they had learnt at school or as adults, a point quite quickly came when the children's knowledge overtook theirs. Susanne's German mother and father (who was a church minister) *'... got to speak very good English, they both did university degrees here, but I remember that my father, if he was doing a sermon in English, he would ask us to check it for him'.*

Parents Who Made Mistakes When Speaking in the Majority Language

Several interviewees remembered as children hearing their parents making mistakes when speaking the majority language. Some mistakes were very basic; others were very subtle distinctions or problems with pronunciation. Interviewees' reactions to them varied widely. Sometimes this was a cause of tension in the family, and some interviewees felt uncomfortable with this. For example, Camilla, the child of Danish parents living in England who spoke good English commented: *'I am still aware at work – because I am a sub-editor – that I get some expressions wrong, e.g. I thought that it was "a hare's breath" and not "a hair's breadth". I can see my Mum does that, she says some of the things that I say … certain things that she says are not quite right. Now, it's quite endearing, but I can see as a child, you want to get it right and that's what I wanted to do'.*

When this happened, some children corrected their parents, which caused tension. After the family moved from Quebec in Canada to Atlanta, for example, Isabelle's mother, whose first language was French, needed to speak English in the community for the first time, and Isabelle was conscious of her mother's mistakes and accent. *'She would sometimes get things wrong, or it was the accent … she would not get the right inflection on something, so I would correct her. Because for me it was wrong and it was embarrassing that my mother would not be saying that word right. But she took it as "Who are you to be correcting me?" It caused a lot of tension'.*

Another interviewee remembers that her reaction to her mother's mistakes changed over time; as a teenager Saadia remembers being embarrassed by mistakes that her mother made in English, although she thinks that as a younger child it did not embarrass her, and that this was part of the common sensitivity that teenagers can have about their parents.

Others were very relaxed. Saad is the son of a Kurdish man who was a professor in Iraq who spoke fluent Arabic to a very high-level, and a Kurdish woman who spoke very limited Arabic. From quite an early age, Saad's Arabic was better than his mother's was. She had a strong Kurdish accent and made a lot of grammatical mistakes. Arabic uses different forms when addressing men and women, and Saad's mother would get this wrong and address men as if they were women and vice versa (which is a particularly embarrassing kind of mistake in this culture). Saad and his siblings would laugh at this and correct her. People understood her but sometimes would make fun of her. She just laughed it off and carried on. Saad does not ever remember being embarrassed by his mother's mistakes.

If your children are likely to hear you speaking a language that you are not fluent in, then you may want to make jokes about any mistakes that you may make, before your children actually pick up on them. Certainly our interviewees suggested that you try to move away from any suggestion of perfectionism around language or embarrassment about any mistakes.

One interviewee, Ingrid, felt that although her widowed American mother living in Sweden was fluent in Swedish, she was not fully aware of all of Swedish culture, traditions, and politics. This may be clearer to Ingrid because she can compare the periods before and after her Swedish father died (when she was 11 years old). Ingrid feels that her father's death meant that she was not exposed to aspects of Swedish culture – her mother did not read a Swedish paper and did not follow Swedish politics. Thus Ingrid notices that her (monolingual) Swedish husband knows far more about politicians, celebrities and public figures than she does. Although her paternal grandparents and relatives did provide some Swedish cultural input, Ingrid still feels that this was less than would have been the case had her father still been there throughout her adolescence. *'When you grow up in a country that is yours, you sort of know who's who … I feel there I've missed out … when I graduated from high school in the States, my mum could tell me about the cap and gown and it was very much like her graduation, but when I graduated from high school in Sweden, my mother had to ask my friends' parents "How do we do this, what are the traditions?"'*

Interviewees Acting as Interpreters for Parents

Although many parents did learn the majority language over time, there were a number of cases where this did not occur and the parents' knowledge of the majority language remained very limited. In several of the families, even many years after they had migrated, the parents' knowledge of the majority language was insufficient to allow them to understand or take part in a conversation (e.g. between the children, see Antony p.69, and a discussion of families with no common language on p.182). In these families, interviewees were often asked to translate between their parents and the outside world, to read letters and fill in forms. These could be occasions that showed the interviewees the value of their bilingualism: Saadia remembers translating a lot for her parents at doctor's and other official appointments, and her parents being very appreciative that the children communicated well in English.

For others, though, there was a sense of awkwardness or regret. Fatima, for instance, said: *'My parents couldn't read or speak English, they spoke Arabic but they didn't read or write Arabic. They were sent to work aged 10, they didn't go to school. We ended up being the children but the translators as well. We were reading the letters. We were a bit embarrassed. I think that if they had had an education, they would have been able to learn more English'.*

One interviewee commented that she sometimes wished that more English had been spoken in the household (rather than Punjabi), as this might have forced her parents to learn to speak (or at least understand) more English: *'Sometimes I feel that if we [the children] had replied in English, it would have forced them to adapt and they would have had to learn better English'.*

Conclusion

- Do not assume children will retain a language that they already speak before moving. They will lose it very quickly unless they receive continued input.

- Interviewees who moved at all ages adjusted well to life in a new country and in a new language. That said, it was certainly a 'bigger deal' for children older than around six years old at the time of the move.
- Children who were born and lived in one setting all their lives who were the children or grandchildren of migrants were not immune from feeling, at times, that they did not fully belong. Most did not, but a few did feel this way.
- If you do not speak the majority language well, be aware that your children will speak it better than you do very quickly and they will be aware of your mistakes and may correct you. If you find this difficult, remember that your child is trying to be helpful, not critical.
- Try to laugh about any mistakes that you make and try not to be embarrassed. If you are in this situation, try to convey to your children from the earliest moments that it is more important to be able to get your message across than to speak the language perfectly. One important way that this message is conveyed is how you prioritise between correct grammar and conveying meaning when your child speaks themselves. So, the advice given to parents when their children make grammatical errors (whether in a monolingual or bilingual family) is to repeat the phrase to the child with the correct grammar – and allow the conversation to move on. Provided that you have been able to understand what the child was trying to say, it is significant that the advice is *not* to ask the child to repeat the phrase correctly. This sends the message that the most important thing was that you understood what your child was trying to say (but that it would be nice if the grammar was also correct). Many of us would welcome it if our children did speak a home language perfectly, but if you are part of a family where either or both parents are using languages learnt in school or as adults imperfectly themselves (whether day-to-day or on holiday with the family), insisting on this is probably unwise.
- Be aware that a child who has been relaxed about an accent or mistakes may nonetheless change their attitude (almost certainly temporarily) in their teenage years.
- Be aware that a child who is desperate to fit in (possibly a child who is shy and does not want to stick out or be noticed for any reason, positive or negative) may be hypersensitive to very minor language mistakes by a parent. He or she might not want a parent to attend events in school because of this. Some would say that you should educate your child to be proud of being different. But this might be easier said than done with a child who is very shy or otherwise desperately wants to 'fit in'. Check that there is no bullying or casual racism going on. Clearly you cannot acquire a perfect knowledge of a second language. You can try pointing out to your child how many other parents speak other languages and that many people speak with slightly different native and non-native accents, and use different phrases and idioms. Ensuring your child has a peer group of children who speak your language can also help – if possible, try to ensure that your child associates these people and the language with very positive experiences.

- Some interviewees felt that they were less plugged into society and less aware of popular figures, politicians and cultural reference points because of their migrant parents. It might be that, if you need advice about how things are done where you live, you can find this out without involving your children or without them overhearing. You might choose to discuss the news or popular books or TV shows with your child. Or you might make a point of family friends passing on their traditions to your children so that they have opportunities to feel part of a long tradition of the majority culture where they live as well as their heritage culture.
- If you possibly can, learn the majority language where you are now living.

3 Interviewees who are Bilingual Solely through Attending School in Another Language

Seven interviewees are included in this group. They vary from a child of an Italian/American father and British mother who attended German- and French-speaking private schools in Switzerland, a Croatian child who attended an Italian school in Croatia, a Kenyan-Asian educated in English in Kenya in the 1930s and interviewees in Argentina, Nigeria and Ghana who were all sent to English-medium or bilingual schools more recently. There are two other cases where children were educated in a language other than their home language, but in both cases this was in multilingual settings and was not the parents' choice, but was due to the language policies of that country. One key distinction between this group and most of our other interviewees is that the school language is not the main majority language, which means that the language is learnt solely through classroom interactions – rather than through day-to-day life, which may subtly affect what is learnt.

Reasons for Choosing a Bilingual/Second Language School

The parents' reasons for sending their children to these schools varied widely. In one case, it was a very pragmatic decision that had nothing to do with the language spoken at the school. Snjezana was enrolled in an Italian school in Croatia mainly because their schedule could be matched with Snjezana's parents' work shifts. The Italian school existed primarily to serve the needs of the 5000 Italian-speaking households in the area. The school was free and run by the state (although there was also some support from the Italian government); all of the lessons were taught in Italian and Croatian was taught as a foreign language. Snjezana had no knowledge of Italian when she started school aged six and neither did 16 out of 20 children in her class.

Other parents chose the schools because they provided a high quality education: Emilio went to a (private) bilingual English/Spanish school in Buenos Aires. He thinks that he was sent to the school because it was a good school, rather than due to any conscious decision by his mother to try to make sure that he learnt English.

In other cases, parents selected schools that taught in a language other than that used at home because they felt that this would give their children advantages later on. Velji, a Kenyan-Asian growing up in Mombasa speaking primarily Gujarati at home in the 1930s and 1940s, attended a school especially for Asian boys in Mombasa. Here all the teaching was carried out in English. Neither of his parents spoke English, but Velji's older sister and brother would help with his homework if he needed help. In turn, Velji's daughter, Bindi, whose first language growing up in Kenya was Gujarati, believes that her parents chose the English-medium school deliberately, although there was probably a Gujarati option, because they felt that it was very important that their children had very good English, as they hoped that their children would go to university in the UK later in their lives.

How were Bilingual Schools Organised?

In most cases, the schools were aware that many of their pupils did not speak the language to be used at the school at all when they started, and the schools were set up to help the children gradually learn the language involved: in Argentina, Emilio, who spoke only Spanish at home, started in the kindergarten aged around three, where Spanish was predominantly used, although the teachers also started to introduce a small amount of English. Emilio thinks that he learnt to read first in Spanish and that reading in English was introduced later. He remembers reading books in English that he thinks would be designed for five year olds when he was seven. From age six, in primary school, half the school day was in English and half was in Spanish.

At Adeyinka's English-medium school in Nigeria, the children were taught to read in English but teachers used Yoruba as a medium to explain things: *'They would say "A is for Apple, B is for Ball and C is for Cat" but then the teacher would add several sentences explaining in more detail in Yoruba. Similarly they would say "add 2 + 4" but the next sentences would be in Yoruba explaining it'*.

Both of these two schools had bilingual staff. Others did not. When the children involved had no knowledge of the language, this was more of an issue. Neither of Snjezana's parents spoke any Italian and she had no knowledge of the language at all when she started school. At her Italian-medium school all the lessons were in Italian from the start, and in addition there was no language support for the 16 children in her class of 20 who did not speak Italian.

In comparison, although when Bindi started school in Kenya the nursery staff did not speak Gujarati, Bindi does not recall any problems being understood in English at nursery and believes that her parents had taught her enough English before she went so that she could understand and make herself understood.

School Rules About Language Use

In many cases, these schools seemed very aware that their pupils had another common language which they could (and might prefer to) communicate in, so many of these schools imposed very strict rules about the language that should be spoken at school. In Snjezana's Italian-medium school in Croatia, speaking Croatian was banned and students were told off if they spoke it between themselves. In Daniela's French-medium boarding school in Switzerland, attended by many international pupils: *'If we were caught speaking our own language we had to pay a fine [taken from their weekly pocket money], so we had to read in French, we had to study in French, it was quite strict, but it helped me learn French quite quickly!'* Daniela even had to write letters home from school to her mother in French, even though her (British) mother understood minimal French.

Adeyinka also mentions that when he went to a boarding secondary school (aged 11) the students were only supposed to speak English. Lessons were now exclusively in English and students had to respond in English. Students who were caught speaking Yoruba to each other were reported and punished.

In fact one of the interviewees who remembers the most severe punishments for speaking a banned language at school is not in this group, although clearly similar issues arise. Pedro grew up in a bilingual family in Texas, in the United States. Despite the fact that most children spoke both English and Spanish at home, the school had a very strict English-only policy: *'Anywhere in the school grounds you could not speak Spanish. ...They'd give you a detention. I got a paddling [beating] many times for speaking Spanish. ... I was always a rebel. I spoke Spanish. You can't tell me not to speak Spanish'.*

Other schools insisted on one language in the classroom but were relaxed about the language that children spoke outside of the classroom. In Kenya, Bindi says, *'As long as in the classroom the teaching medium was English, there wasn't a strong negative reaction to speaking any other language outside the classroom'.* Despite this, Bindi says, *'We played in English, the playground language was English'* which may have been because the children attending the school were very mixed, with Kenyan-Asians and those speaking several different Kenyan languages all at the same school.

In other schools, although there may not have been punishments, speaking the required language consistently and accurately in class was essential to do well. At Emilio's English-medium school in Argentina, during the afternoons the teachers spoke only English and the children were supposed to reply in English. Sometimes the children would not understand and would reply in Spanish, but the teachers would insist that the children spoke English, and the teachers would say, *'Say it in English, say it in English'.* Children who continued to reply in Spanish did not get good marks.

Some Possible Downsides

Emilio, who attended a bilingual English/Spanish school in Argentina, commented on the way this bilingual schooling was organised. From age six in primary school, half the school day was in English and half was in Spanish. The children were taught English grammar rules and spelling as well as teaching through immersion. The school tended to repeat subjects in both languages, so they studied history in Spanish, which focused on Argentinean and world history. They then did history again in the afternoon in English, when they covered English or European history. Emilio remembers learning about Stonehenge and the kings and queens of England. (He points out that the content of the lessons was partly dictated by the materials available.) Possibly because of this doubling up of subjects, school ran from 8am until 5pm but the children also had homework (in English or Spanish), which would take them another hour to do.

In Emilio's case, the school switched to using Spanish as the sole teaching medium when he was 11 years old. The children now studied English only a few hours a week, and Emilio feels that he made much less progress in English after this point. However, he did retain his English and was able to use it during a visit to the United States and in the UK where he studied for an MA. However, he points out that, probably because of this reduction of input, this did not apply to everybody. Thus *'of the students in my class, I reckon only half have a level of English that they can use today'*.

Although some of these children at times saw downsides to the educational choices made by their parents, they all felt that they had ultimately benefitted from their education in another language. Emilio, for example, says, *'We all pretty much saw it as a burden, to be honest, … what a drag … but then later on (maybe when I was 10) I enjoyed reading books in English … books like* Lord of the Flies, Oliver Twist, An Inspector Calls …*'.*

In Snjezana's case, the downsides were to do with the fact that the school clearly preferred children from the Italian community in Croatia who spoke Italian at home: Snjezana also feels that the school was very discriminatory. *'I actually had a situation when all my marks in Italian language and literacy were the highest, but when the final grades were awarded, I did not get the highest grade. And the explanation given was that I was not a native Italian speaker'.* Numerous similar examples over the years demonstrated that mother tongue Italian speakers were given preference and were valued over and above those students who spoke only Croatian at home – regardless of their work or attainment at school. Snjezana remembers one (Italian-speaking) parent being concerned that the non-Italian-speaking children would hold the Italian-speaking ones back (although this was not the case at all).

Was There Any Support for the School Language in the Community?

Interviewees varied in the amount of input or interaction in the language of their schooling outside of school. In Emilio's case, although he spoke English at school, he never had a conversation in English outside of school until he was 16 or 17, and he did not visit an English-speaking country until he was 18. (Although his sisters were also attending bilingual schools they never spoke English at home.) Outside school, however, Emilio did see films in English and listened to music with English lyrics: *'It was cool to know the words of a song in English. My parents or my family always told me that English would be useful later when I grew up, but as a kid, I didn't care. But knowing the songs and being able to understand a movie in the original language was an immediate plus'.*

Similarly, Adeyinka commented that in Nigeria at this time there were new radio stations broadcasting in English. Everyone wanted to listen to the new music that they were playing. *'People now started to imitate these English, English, English things …. You had to be sophisticated and listen to English programmes and English music'.*

Gaps in the Vocabulary Learnt at School

One other point was made by two interviewees concerning the limitations of learning a language solely through school (and these were the interviewees whose parents spoke none or very little of the school's language). Both Snjezana and Emilio reported that there were gaps in their vocabulary such as the names of simple household implements. Snjezana says, '*So, for instance, how do you say "colander" in Italian? I had no idea. The fact that you were unable to say "colander" in Italian made your language less worthy [at school]'*. While in Emilio's case, despite the good level of English that he achieved through attending bilingual school, he is aware that there were lots of household objects for which he did not know the words in English and he only learnt these when he moved to London.

Snjezana adds to this when she says: '*Even now I feel that some of my knowledge is compartmentalised in languages. Some things I have learnt in some languages …. I have never studied in Croatian … and some terminology is missing'*.

Snjezana raised one other issue that arose from her education in a second language, which is that she feels sensitive about making mistakes when she speaks in a language that she does not speak fluently – and she attributes this to be being corrected or made fun of at school. This has made her reluctant to speak languages she knows less well as this would put her in the position of potentially making mistakes. She says, '*I will choose the language based on the ones I speak best, rather than what is best suited to the occasion'*.

All our interviewees who went to a school that operated in a language that they did not speak elsewhere – neither at home nor in the community – ended up speaking that language fluently. Some attended school for as little as three years, but with some additional input thereafter maintained the language. Nevertheless, Emilio tells us about his classmates who studied half of their time in English from age six to age 11, but with input reduced to a few hours a week after that point, and very limited or no input since, have now lost their English and they would not be able to speak it today.

Interviewees Sent to a Second Language School Because of a National Language Policy

There were also three cases of interviewees growing up in multilingual countries where the policy of the country was that children were educated in a language that few families spoke at home. These were Aimee in Togo who spoke Kabye at home, Mina in the community and French at school; Fatima in Morocco who spoke Arabic at home but attended a bilingual Arabic and French school until she was 10; and Rose in Singapore who spoke Cantonese, Mandarin and Hokkien at home and English at school.

Aimee

In Aimee's case, all schooling was in French while she lived in Togo. The staff at the school were Togolese but were supposed to only speak French. The children were aware that the staff could speak Mina and occasionally the latter would use Mina, for example when disciplining children. There was a national policy that all education would be in French, which the teachers followed. *'In Togo, in class we were not allowed to speak Mina or Kabye and you were beaten if you did. In the playground, we spoke Mina, although I had some friends who spoke Kabye as well'*. After leaving Togo to live in France with her aunt when she was eight, Aimee continued to study in French (the majority language) and to speak Kabye at home. (For more on this transition, see p.49 and p.119.)

Fatima

In Fatima's case, her primary school, like all schools in Morocco, was bilingual. In the morning all lessons were in Arabic, and in the afternoon all lessons were in French. By the age of 10, Fatima's French was good: *'Because it is really hammered into you, … three or four hours a day, solid French …maths, history whatever …'.*

When she was 10, Fatima left Morocco to come to join her parents in the UK where she did the normal French as a second language classes with all the other children, she says: *'I was **very** good at French … I would always show off, because I spoke French and I knew what the teacher was saying and I had learnt to write it …'.* Despite having no other input in French other than these second language classes, Fatima did not lose her French and is still comfortable speaking it today, although she has few opportunities to do so.

Rose

In Rose's case, her parents separated when she was young and she spent time living with both of them. Her father spoke Cantonese but not Mandarin. Her mother started off speaking Cantonese to her, but then switched first to Mandarin and then to English (as she was trying to learn this language herself). During each school term Rose stayed with her godmother who spoke Hokkien to her. The Singaporean authorities introduced a 'speak English campaign'. This meant that at school every subject was taught in English, apart from Mandarin, which was taught as a subject. The children also continued to speak some Mandarin amongst themselves. The children had incentives to speak English: *'In one class even, the teacher got us to pay 10 pence into a piggy bank for every time we spoke any other language than English, and at the end of the month the teacher would buy sweeties for the class'.* In fact, this language policy went beyond school and many in Singapore started to use English at home – as did Rose's mother. Rose says as a result, *'Now everyone speaks English in Singapore, it's almost like in India'.* She herself feels that English is her strongest language because of this education in English, although she sees Cantonese as her first language – and she prefers doing maths in Mandarin. Subsequently, the government also introduced a 'Speak Mandarin Campaign – don't forget your roots'. Rose attributes the reversal of government language policy to the economic opening up of China, which was a significant opportunity for Singapore but which required good Mandarin language skills. Rose feels that in Singapore people are confused; before they were told to speak English, now they are also told to speak Mandarin. Because of this confusion, she feels that many people in Singapore are left speaking no language particularly well. She feels that there is a particular problem with accents and pronunciation. However she also points out that during the 'Speak English' campaign the main input for many children in Mandarin was through Mandarin teachers who she feels *are boring, not very interactive and only give out vocabulary and then test it the following week'.*

Conclusion

- If you enrol your child in a school using a medium that they do not already speak, make sure that some kind of language support will be available or liaise with the school to see what you can put in place from home.
- Be aware that some schools in some settings may have a strong preference for children who are mother tongue speakers of the language.
- Be prepared for schools to have strict rules about what languages are spoken – certainly in the classroom, but possibly also during breaks.
- Children who learn a language solely through schooling may feel that they have particular gaps in their vocabulary. For example, they may feel that they do not know the words for household objects in their school language (e.g. colander, bathmat), but that equally they do not know words most frequently learnt in school in their home language (e.g. words for long division or historical periods or scientific terms).
- Children who learn a language through schooling are particularly vulnerable to losing it when they leave school or change schools because they are more likely to have learnt it in isolation with no input from elsewhere.
- Songs, films, books, TV and radio broadcasts in a language learnt mainly or solely at school can help introduce different sorts of vocabulary and usage. Our interviewees suggested that where these were considered high status or 'cool' amongst the children involved, they also helped support the children's motivation to learn that language.

4 Interviewees who Learnt Languages Solely from the Community

Quite a few interviewees mentioned learning a language from neighbours and from the community even when this was the sole input. Some were exposed to it over long periods of time, and others seem to have learnt languages very quickly. Some subsequently lost all or part of the language afterwards, however.

Aimee

For example, there are 40 dialects or local languages spoken in Togo where Aimee was born. Both her parents were from the northern Kabye tribe and they spoke the Kabye language. However, she was brought up in the south as her parents were working in the capital city of the country where most people spoke Mina. At home she spoke Kabye, whereas with the family's neighbours and friends she spoke Mina. (In class, as described on p.42, she spoke French.) Aimee's mother and father spoke Kabye together at home. Aimee remembers that her parents wanted her to learn Kabye and to feel that she belonged to this tribe. Despite this she does not remember any particular pressure to speak any of the three languages: she just felt that it was natural to do this. She explains that most people in Togo are multilingual as it is a relatively small country and people from different groups learn each other's languages through interaction on a daily basis. However, Aimee moved to France to live with an aunt when she was eight after her parents' divorce. After this point she no longer had any input in Mina and lost her knowledge of the language fairly rapidly.

Matilde

One interviewee living where several languages were spoken locally learnt the international language rather than the community's first language. Matilde is Italian and lived in a very remote region of what was then Zaire for two years from when she was six years old (the fact that there was no school confirms just how remote it was). She told us that there was a local language, Mashi, but many in the community also spoke French because Zaire had been a Belgian colony. Matilde's parents spoke French but spoke only Italian to her at home and between themselves. The family had a nanny/ home help who spoke French to the children and who did not speak Italian, so conversations between her and Matilde's mother would also be in French. As there was no school, Matilde studied at home with her mother. Within this two-year period Matilde learnt to speak French from playing with other children in the village, as well as perhaps from the nanny/home help. She comments that French was not, in fact, the first language of the children that she played with – that was the local language, Mashi. It was perhaps strange that she learnt French and not Mashi. But by the end of the two-year stay, she could communicate easily in French.

Charles

One interviewee did learn the majority language solely from 'the streets', but he is not very confident speaking it without making mistakes today. Charles was born and raised in Luxembourg. His father was a bilingual French and Luxembourgian speaker, but decided to speak French to his children. Charles was also educated in French. Charles learnt Luxembourgian in the streets, while speaking to other people and kids in Luxembourg, but he never had any formal education in Luxembourgian. He understands Luxembourgian very well today, but cannot speak it that much. He was also exposed to it when he went to a boarding school in Belgium where most pupils were Luxembourgian, but even with them he spoke mostly in French. *'The only time that I really used Luxembourgian was when I was doing my PhD. I was doing my research about Luxembourg and I was analysing parliamentary debates and policy data in French and Luxembourgian. It came back much, much later in life. … When I activated Luxembourgian, I felt "ohhh this is tough", and I am glad I speak German as well because there are so many similarities. I had to have a dictionary with me all the time because of the terminology, which was more than just "street Luxembourgian!"'*

Privately, when he is in Luxembourg with friends and so on, Charles speaks French. Whenever he needs to deal with any administrative matters in Luxembourg (like getting an ID card), Charles makes an effort to speak Luxembourgian so he is not treated as a foreigner, although French is one of the official languages. *'I might make mistakes when I speak it, but I know I will get treated better than if I speak French'.*

Others who learnt a language in a similar way have still retained it. Josune grew up hearing only Basque at home from her extended family who all lived together. The family spoke only Basque at home and Josune also attended a Basque school where all lessons were in Basque, apart from a weekly Spanish lesson. However, she heard Spanish from the TV (as there was no TV in Basque at this time). As she lived in a city she feels that she had more opportunities to hear and speak Spanish than she would have had if she had grown up in the countryside. Outside school she also mixed with some children who only spoke Spanish, and as they got older, even in school, Josune and her friends started to speak more Spanish. Josune still speaks Spanish fluently today.

Armelle, who had spoken French and Spanish at home and at school, reported having learnt a language from the community extremely quickly. When she was seven and the family moved to Italy, Armelle again went to an international French school, but she says that she picked up Italian very quickly within a month – from the playground, the TV and the community, and she still speaks Italian fluently today.

Velji

A very interesting example of interviewees learning languages solely from the community is Velji, the child of Gujarati-speaking Kenyan-Asians, who was born in Mombasa in 1933. It was Velji's grandparents who had left India to come to Kenya, and so he was a third-generation migrant. His family still spoke Gujarati exclusively at home. Although the majority of the local population were Swahili speakers, there was a large Gujarati-speaking population in the area which Velji and his family mixed with. They would go to a temple where Gujarati was spoken. The language used in shops was Gujarati (or other Asian languages and dialects), as most shops were owned by Kenyan Asians, whereas in the fruit and vegetable market the main language used would be Swahili. At this time Kenya was a British colony, and the authorities had established special schools for Kenyan-Asian children where the medium of education was English. In these schools, Swahili was not used as a medium of education, nor was it taught as a language. Most children growing up in Asian households at this time did not learn any significant Swahili – neither Velji's brother nor his sister did so. However, Velji was a very keen football player and he went out often to play football with other children in Mombasa, and this led him to learn to speak both Swahili and other dialects of Gujarati. Velji explains that his older sister and brother did not go out and play with the other children in this way, and so they became bilingual in Gujarati and English, but did not learn Swahili or the other dialects of Gujarati.

Velji was able to build on his knowledge learnt from the community when he passed his exams and left school aged 16 and got a job working for British American Tobacco (BAT). For many years, part of his job involved travelling along the coast of Kenya and Tanzania checking on the sales of BAT products. This enabled him to learn other dialects of both Swahili and Gujarati. He also taught himself to read Swahili during this time; he explains that Swahili is written in roman script and so he found it relatively easy to read letters from his Swahili-speaking suppliers and so on.

Velji's childhood passion for football ensured that he interacted with the Swahili-speaking community, whereas his brothers, sisters and peers did not. This equipped him not only for his work at BAT, where his languages meant that he was given extra responsibilities and gained promotions, but also for a subsequent career as an interpreter and translator for the courts, police and the Home Office in the UK. In particular, Velji's relatively unusual intimate knowledge of the different dialects of Swahili spoken up and down the coasts of Kenya and Tanzania has proved extremely useful to these authorities.

Conclusion

- Children can learn a language solely from interacting with the community (e.g. when the language is not spoken at home or at school). Some children have done so relatively quickly.

- Some children later lost this language when there was no longer any input, but others did not.
- Language learnt in this way is likely to have some gaps, but can be a strong basis that can be built on if the language is used in later life.
- Learning a language in this way will depend on how much time a child spends in the community – just being in a community and being surrounded by a language is not enough. There needs to be a significant amount of interaction in that language. We are also aware of other instances where children did not learn a majority language (e.g. a child in a wealthy family growing up in Pakistan who spoke English at home and at school and who gained quite a limited knowledge of Urdu from the community).
- In a bilingual community, you may find that most people will speak to visitors or migrants into the community in a language seen as more appropriate to outsiders, an international language rather than a more locally spoken one.

5 Changes as a Result of Divorce or Separation

Six of our interviewees had parents who divorced or separated while they were growing up. Although the impact of this on the interviewees overall was probably always significant, if we look solely at the impact on the interviewees' languages, in some cases this seemed to be relatively minor. This was particularly true when the divorce happened when the children were very young, if both parents remained in the same area and the children remained in contact with both of them. Interviewees reported a more significant impact when the parents moved to different countries after the divorce (which was more likely if they had different origins or nationalities). In fact, the main impact on interviewees stemmed from the changes of circumstances, particularly as in some cases divorces prompted changes of country as well as changes in terms of who interviewees interacted with on a daily basis. Examples of low-levels of impact resulting from divorce included Rose. Her Singaporean parents divorced but she continued to see both her father, who spoke to her only in Cantonese, and her mother, who spoke at different times Cantonese, Mandarin or English. The divorce was not a factor in her bilingual childhood, whilst Singapore's language policy certainly was (see also p.43). Charles's parents separated, but as both were speaking to him in French by this time (his father had never used Luxembourgian to his children and his mother had started off speaking Dutch but switched to French), this did not affect the languages he used at all.

Aimee

In other cases, however, the divorce did impact on the languages that the interviewees spoke as well as on the environment they lived in. We have already briefly referred to (p.42) Aimee's move from Togo to France to live with her aunt when she was eight, which was prompted by her parents' divorce. Had her father's sister been living in Togo the impact on Aimee may well have been negligible, but the fact that she moved to live with her aunt in France meant that the consequences of the divorce were significant on her use of languages. In Togo, Aimee was speaking French, Kabye and Mina. In France she neither heard nor spoke Mina and she quickly lost this language. She did continue to speak French and Kabye, but the pattern in terms of where she spoke each language was reversed. In Togo she spoke Kabye at home, Kabye and Mina in the community and French at school, whereas in France she spoke French at school and in the community, and Kabye at home with her aunt's family. In France, her aunt was married to another Kabye speaker, and she had six children of her own. As long as she lived with her aunt, she feels that she sustained her Kabye to quite a high-level (although her father had a different view, see below). Certainly since leaving France and her aunt's household (Aimee now lives in London), she is aware that her Kabye has deteriorated. She commented that ostensibly her father mainly cared that his children had a good education in French. But every summer when the children went to visit, it was important that they took part in traditional ceremonies, for which the Kabye language was essential. After a while, even during the period when Aimee was still living with her aunt and speaking Kabye at home, her father felt that her Kabye was getting less fluent. This was important to him because he wanted the whole family to be able to participate in the traditional ceremonies.

Daniela

Another example where a divorce had far-reaching consequences was Daniela. Her Italian-American father and British mother divorced when she was almost four. The family had been living in Italy at the time, and Daniela's mother moved back to Hertfordshire in England. Daniela believes that while they lived in Italy her mother spoke both Italian and English to her. Certainly when she and her mother came to England and her mother hired a British nanny to look after her Daniela spoke only Italian to the nanny who could not understand her. Daniela's mother switched to speaking to her only in English in an attempt to fit in with English village life. Daniela's mother did want her to stay in contact with her father, and Italian was not totally essential for this because her father spoke fluent English (as well as six other languages). When Daniela visited him in Italy after the divorce, she spoke English to him but he would speak to her in both French and Italian: *'He was* **very** *keen to get me back into speaking Italian'*. It helped that Daniela had grandparents and cousins in Italy who were always speaking Italian around her when she was a small child. Also, in order to motivate her to learn Italian, her father used to buy Daniela her favourite comics in Italian (Asterix and Obelix), and this motivated her to read them in Italian. She would ask him for help if she could not understand some words.

When she was eight, Daniela went to a French-medium boarding school in Switzerland, and after this she increasingly spoke to her father in French as well. At this point, her father used to travel from Italy to Switzerland to visit her and she saw him more often than she saw her mother. Her Italian cousins also spoke French and the mixing of languages was very normal: *'If you could not think of a word in one language, you would use a word in another language. I just kind of accepted that's what it was like when I was with my Italian family. That was normal to me. My French took over from my Italian and sometimes my cousins would tease me about my Italian and they would say "You are very English when you speak Italian!"'*

Two years later (from when Daniela was 10 until she was 14) there was a four- year period when Daniela did not see her father and only spoke to him occasionally over the phone. During these phone calls they would speak in English or French. She did not use any Italian during this time and now feels that this four-year gap was critical. When her father moved to France she started to visit him from the age of 14 and they spoke only in French. Now Daniela says: *'My French is much more fluent than my Italian, oddly enough, even though I would class it as my third language [i.e. in the order she learnt it], it's my second language [i.e. in terms of how well she speaks it]. I kept my French up much more, and I think partly because French is a more useful language universally.... so it's been a really good language to have for communicating with other people'.* (For more on Daniela using Italian more recently see p.163.)

In Christopher's case, the impact of divorce on the languages he heard and spoke was minimal because he attended a French-medium school. He spoke French to his mother and English to his father who separated when he was 10. Christopher lived with his father after this point and his home language became English. Fortunately, for his bilingualism at least, at this time he was attending the French-medium *lycée* (school) in London, which meant that he was hearing and speaking almost exclusively French at school. However, he did tell us that because his mother left the family, he felt that there was a barrier between him and his mother at times, and that he felt more at home with his father. Christopher was one of the interviewees who had decided not to raise his children bilingually, and it is tempting to wonder whether he might have reached a different decision had his parents not divorced.

Isabelle

The interviewee whose bilingual childhood was most affected by divorce was Isabelle, the child of a French mother and a Polish-Canadian father living in Quebec City, in Canada. Her father opted to speak English to her, her mother spoke French and she learnt some Polish from her grandparents (see p.26). The family moved to Atlanta when Isabelle was six, where she attended a bilingual programme in a French-medium school. After three years in Atlanta, when Isabelle was nine and a half, her parents separated. This was not an amicable separation and the relationship between her parents was very tense. Isabelle moved together with her mother and younger brother to Paris. Already upset by her parents' separation, she did not want to move at all. She had visited Paris once with her parents and had enjoyed staying with and playing with her cousins, but nonetheless she felt that she was moving to a strange country which she did not know. *'I didn't want to go. I had just started to make friends ... And then we left. I was really upset. I didn't want to go to this place that I felt I didn't know at all ... my mother's family that I had met maybe a couple of times ...'.*

In Paris, Isabelle was suddenly in an almost totally French environment – she spoke French with her mother and went to a normal French state school. She did, however, consciously decide to continue to speak English with her brother. *'I really tried. It was the only way to keep it real – whatever my life had been before that. My brother and I had a lot of conflicts growing up, but on this point, we did it, we spoke to each other in English'.*

With the separation and the move, Isabelle's mother also became quite anti-American. For example, she forbade Isabelle from wearing jeans. However, she remained keen that her children should be bilingual – and she did not interfere with them speaking

English together or with Isabelle reading in English. Isabelle did have some other input in English; she wrote to her father each week and he wrote back. (She preferred writing to speaking on the phone although she did phone her father sometimes too.) He sent her English books, and when she was given a radio for Christmas she also started listening to the BBC in English early each morning. Isabelle's mother wanted her children to continue to have a relationship with their father, and there was also a court order specifying that he should have access. Isabelle and her brother visited her father three times a year for holidays (mostly in Atlanta, although a couple of times he came to Europe to see them). Despite her relatively low-level of input in English at this time, she remembers no problem in switching languages for these visits even though the transitions were often fraught for other reasons because of the tension between her parents. However, she does remember: '... *coming back to France and wanting to make the English thing last as long as possible ... to try to stretch it out ... to pretend I wasn't there'.*

When Isabelle was almost 16, she discovered that her father had a potentially fatal illness and she decided that she wanted to go and live with him. She pushed very hard to make this happen, although at the same time she was nervous about implying to her mother that she did not want to live with her. Her father took up an opportunity to take a year of work in Belgium, and both Isabelle and her brother moved to live with him there. They were both enrolled in an international school that had a bilingual English and French stream.

After this transition year, Isabelle and her brother moved back to Atlanta to live with her father. (The transitions between schooling systems are described in Chapter 14, p.117.) Isabelle's experiences seem to an outside observer to have been so difficult that although generally interviewees' feelings about their bilingual childhoods are included in Chapter 19 (p.153), it seems important to me to include here that she says: *'It was great [being raised bilingually]. It was quite complicated because of what happened with my parents. But it is valuable. I think your imaginary world is much richer. You have cultural experiences and cultural references, and so a richer inner life. I've never not had it. ... I had all these problems with my mother, yes, that's true, but that doesn't mean that I hate French. I had very mixed feelings about Paris because I didn't want to be there and I still have mixed feelings about it. But objectively it is a beautiful city and it's an interesting culture and it is part of my culture. I can't pretend it's not, and I won't. It does make me who I am too. It is a gift to be able to understand several languages'.*

Conclusion

Divorce can impact on children in a variety of ways. Here we are thinking – somewhat artificially – only about their bilingualism.

• Given the stresses and strains the family will be under, bilingualism may simply need to be a casualty of divorce. Clearly, where a child's input in one language is solely from one parent, if that parent is no longer living in the family home, the impact on the child's bilingualism might be important. This was certainly the case for Daniela's Italian. In other families, the children will continue to have one language at home and one at school as Christopher did. In other families, the children will spend part of the time with each parent, although if they only spend alternate weekends with (usually) their father, this may not be enough input if their father is the sole source of input in a language. Bear in mind that relationships with grandparents and the wider family are also often vulnerable after a divorce, which will be even more the case if the children are no longer able to speak a common language with their grandparents, aunts, uncles and cousins. And, of course, children may also lose touch with grandparents and wider family who may otherwise been a source of input in a vulnerable language.

- You might be able to arrange schooling or a childminder to replace the input of an absent parent.
- If you are a mixed-language family, it is more likely that one parent will move country after a divorce than is the case for divorcing couples generally, with all the consequences this has on contact between that parent and the children.
- If your children are older, you might be able to enlist the help of an older sibling to continue input in a vulnerable language (although this would be asking quite a lot).

Of the interviewees whose parents divorced, none mentioned that their parents married new partners. Remarriage after divorce is probably more common nowadays, and the impact of stepmothers and step-siblings who do or do not speak a home language could be very important. (For one example of the influence of a stepmother see Sabina's account of her father's remarriage after her mother died, p.55.)

6 Changes as a Result of the Death of One Parent

We interviewed three people whose father or mother died whilst they were children. Emilio's father died when he was very young (not yet three years old). This clearly had a big impact on his family and on him growing up, but it did not impact on his bilingualism because his sole input in his second language was his bilingual school. The other two interviewees lost parents much later and with greater direct impacts on their language environment. One interviewee lost her father when she was 11, and another lost her mother when she was nine. In the second of these, the remaining parent remarried. Clearly, losing a parent when aged nine or 11 is always going to be traumatic for children with far-reaching consequences far beyond the languages they hear and speak, but here we focus particularly on the linguistic aspects of their experience.

Ingrid

Ingrid grew up in a mixed-language family with an American mother and Swedish father living in Sweden until her father died when she was 11 years old. Her mother decided to remain in Sweden (despite the fact that the family had twice previously tried to relocate back to the United States), and Ingrid continued to get English from her mother, Swedish input from school, the community and her Swedish extended family, and maintained her bilingualism. She still felt the loss of her father though. She explains that it meant that she no longer had a parent or other resource who could read and write academic-level Swedish. Ingrid did not have anyone who could read and check her essays or homework before it was handed in and point out any errors. (Her paternal grandparents had stopped school early and could not do this, and her mother's written Swedish was not good enough.) Once or twice she showed her work to her classmates and asked them to do this for her. Unfortunately, one classmate laughed at some spelling mistakes, which must have been very hurtful and clearly made a strong impression on Ingrid who has always had a lingering lack of confidence in her written Swedish as a result. *'Still today, with written Swedish, I am confident with talking and writing things but when I need to show someone ... hand it in to someone who is going to judge it, it gets really difficult for me to part with it ... This fear has stayed with me ... "What if they laugh?"'* As mentioned earlier (see p.35), Ingrid also felt after her father's death that she missed out on Swedish culture and politics, and on having a family member who knew how things worked or how things were done.

Sabina

The death of Sabina's mother when she was nine changed her whole language environment. Sabina was born in the UK; both her parents were from Pakistan and had come to the UK as adults. They had both learnt English but spoke Urdu between themselves. As a child, Sabina and her brother (who is six years older than her) were raised speaking Urdu at home. Sabina picked up English from going to nursery and then to school. Sabina continued to speak Urdu with both her parents until her mother died when she was nine. *'I don't know why but at this time I started speaking English to my Dad. I can't pinpoint why I did that. Was it just because my Mum had died? Or was it because of my age? I don't know'.* Sabina thinks that from this point in time her father also replied to her (at least often, if not consistently) in English and, as a result, for a while the Urdu input in her life was minimal. She does not remember any attempts on her father's part to get her to continue to speak Urdu. (Clearly this would have been a very difficult time for the whole family who were grieving and her father who was having to cope with being a single parent.) A couple of years after her mother died, Sabina's father remarried. Sabina refers to her father's second wife as her 'second mother'. She came from Pakistan to marry Sabina's father, did not speak a word of English and also refused to learn it in spite of Sabina's efforts to teach her. (Sabina was concerned that her second mother would not even be able to make a 999 call or ask for any kind of help if there was ever an emergency.) Sabina explains that her second mother had left a close and extended family behind in Pakistan to marry Sabina's father, had not really wanted to leave Pakistan and had found it hard to adjust to life in the UK. This context may explain her second mother's determination not to learn English. Sabina comments, *'So then in a way I had to relearn Urdu because by that time I was speaking English all the time. ... It was quite hard [to go back to speaking Urdu]'.* Sabina did regain fluent spoken Urdu (with a slight accent) and is totally confident speaking Urdu in social situations. Sabina had no choice but to speak Urdu to her second mother, but remembers continuing to speak mainly English with her father until she was an adult.

Conclusion

- Given the stresses and strains the family will be under, bilingualism may simply need to be a casualty of bereavement. Clearly where a child's input in one language is solely from one parent, and that parent has died, the impact on the child's bilingualism will be significant. In other families, the children will continue to have one language at home and one at school and in the community, as Ingrid did.
- If you are a mixed-language family, you might be able to arrange schooling or a childminder to replace the input in one language.
- Bear in mind that the children may also miss the cultural input, local knowledge, and support with homework and academic work of a mother tongue or very fluent parent who is now absent. See what you can do to arrange suitable substitutes

from family, neighbours or friends, or diligently help them with spellcheckers, dictionaries and grammar books.

- Remember that Sabina switched to the majority language after her mother died. If your children do suddenly develop resistance to speaking one language, do continue speaking to them in that language so that they retain a passive knowledge (which they may well be able to switch to actively using –see also Chapter 11 on resistance, p.81).

7 Changes as a Result of Advice Given to Parents

In most cases, the advice given to parents was as I would expect based on my experience at WFBG drop-in events and my reading in this subject area: 'Speak your first or most fluent language to your child' or variations of this. However, there was one unfortunate exception.

Christine

Christine was the child of a German mother and French father living in France. At around the time that Christine started school (between the ages of four and six), her mother was advised to stop speaking German to her. *'She was advised that speaking two languages would be confusing'*. This was despite the fact that Christine's French was at native level and she was fluent and had a wide vocabulary and good grammar for her age. Christine remembers discussing this with her mother some time later (her mother has since died) and was told that, *'I did what I thought was the right thing. People told me that it was going to be confusing for you and so I stopped'*. Christine mentions that her brother, who is three years younger than her, was a late talker and was not saying many clear words at the age of three. (The family story is that he would point and grunt and Christine's mother would know what he wanted and would give it to him. Aged three he was sent to his paternal grandmother for a week, who did not understand his pointing and grunting and he began to talk.) It is possible that because of Christine's brother speaking later than average, her mother was advised that their bilingual situation was at fault and was persuaded to stop speaking German to both her children. It is equally possible that teachers where Christine had started preschool or school intervened and gave her mother the advice.

After this point in time, Christine's mother spoke only French to her. Christine does recall at some point later that there were some attempts to have days when the family would speak only German, but Christine's brother was unable or reluctant to participate in these and they never took off. Christine had few books in German and did not read them. At that time there was no video and no chance of German TV or films, and so Christine's input in German was reduced to the odd word mixed into sentences by her mother for a particularly German object or concept and the time spent with the family during holidays. The family went to stay with relatives in Germany at least once each year and sometimes twice, and would sometimes stay several weeks. Christine did not have cousins, but had uncles who did not speak much French, as well as grandparents who did not speak any French, and so she maintained her German almost entirely through these periodic visits.

Christine is very glad that she is bilingual. *'What is interesting is that we didn't speak German at home much, but our parents were still expecting us to be bilingual ... [laughs]'.* She is in regular touch with her German relatives, most of whom do not speak French or English and who she speaks to in German. *'I think that it is very good in general for learning ... for the brain ... all that flexibility'.* She does regret that her mother did not continue speaking German with her. When she meets German people in England, she tends to speak English with them, partly because they meet in an English-language context and partly because she is now more comfortable speaking English. She rarely watches a German film or reads a book in German and now feels that if her mother had pursued speaking German with her, she would be more likely to access German culture and her German heritage. Christine did spectacularly well to retain her German given the very limited input that she had after the age of around five. Many other children would have lost any ability to speak or understand German.

Conclusion

- Sadly, my conclusion from this needs to be that whatever problems you encounter, whatever advice you seek or are given along the way, think very carefully before you follow advice given to you by a professional who is not specifically trained or experienced in multilingualism. This applies whether the professional is a doctor, teacher, health visitor or even a speech therapist. In particular, provided that your child does not have any disability or any significant behavioural issues and you are speaking a language you speak fluently to your child, think very carefully before following any advice that suggests that you should stop speaking the language that you have always spoken to your child. (Especially, as is more than likely, if the advice is to give up speaking a minority language and start speaking a majority language to your child.)
- Speaking to your child in a language that you do not speak very fluently is much more likely to be damaging to the child than speaking a language you speak fluently or which is your mother tongue.
- Multilingual children will often go through a phase of mixing languages. This is usually short-lived and is perfectly normal. It is not a reason to stop speaking a language to your child. If your child does have a significant speech delay or other problems, it is very unlikely that your multilingual situation has anything to do with this. Altering the languages spoken will almost certainly not help and may confuse the child. If a problem is (incorrectly) attributed to multilingualism, it will mean that no one is looking for or dealing with any other factors.
- Although Christine's example is a couple of decades old, it is still common for bilingual families to be given outdated, ill-founded and unhelpful advice from those who are qualified in other fields but who do not actually know very much about bilingualism. We are aware of recent examples in the UK, and also in France.

- If you are given advice and you are unsure about it, ask for a second opinion from someone with some extra training in bilingualism. This is your right and you should not be embarrassed to ask for this. You may have to do some digging yourself to try to locate the right person. You also may not be able to find this locally – although in the UK in most areas you should be able to. There are now several international websites that focus on multilingual families where you can post questions and get answers from other families as well as specialists (see p.225 for a list of web resources) so if you are given advice and you want an informal second opinion on it, this is a good place to go.
- Sometimes recently trained professionals are better informed about bilingualism, as research and thinking on the issue has changed considerably over the last two decades in some countries, so if there is genuinely not a specialist in bilingualism available, you could also try getting some advice from someone who has trained more recently.
- Remember that this is your family and these are your children and, although it is very hard to go against what a qualified person says is best for your child, advice is just that and you do not need to follow it if you are not comfortable with it.
- If you are given advice by a professional that you feel is substandard, it would be helpful for other parents coming after you if you can find constructive ways to give feedback either to that individual or to his or her team leader or manager so that they can look at some more training for that individual or team. This is particularly important where giving advice to parents on bringing up children or where their language development is central to the professional's role (e.g. in the UK a speech therapist or health visitor) which means that their poor advice is very likely to get repeated to other families.

8 Changes as a Result of Interviewees' Choices or Decisions

The starting point for this book was to examine the assertion that: 'When your children are grown up, they will be glad that you made the effort to raise them bilingually'. This does tend to imply that the key decisions about bilingual childhoods are made by adults, and that the children are relatively passive in this process. Several of our interviewees, though, reminded us that even as quite young children they played a very active, and often a determining role, in deciding whether they would be bilingual and/or which languages they would understand and speak.

In some cases, as with Velji's unusual mixing with Swahili-speaking children (described above, see p.47), this was not about language per se; his knowledge of Swahili was an unsought by-product of his passion for football. Some interviewees did make positive decisions explicitly about retaining languages – so for example (as discussed above, see p.51) Isabelle remembers making a positive and conscious decision at the age of nine to carry on speaking English to her brother when their parents divorced and they moved from the United States to France. However, she suggests that this is partly because she was struggling to come to terms with her parents' divorce and the changes that this brought about in her life, and that her decision was not mainly because she particularly wanted to speak English or to be bilingual. However, some children did make very conscious decisions about speaking more than one language or about learning a particular language.

Sophie

Sophie's adopted grandfather had always spoken some Spanish to her as a young child (for more on her childhood in south-west France speaking French, Occitan and Spanish, see p.25). When Sophie started studying Spanish formally in school when she was 10, she went to this adopted grandfather and asked him to speak Spanish to her more systematically, and he also helped her with her Spanish homework. When she was 15, Sophie went to boarding school because she really wanted to learn Italian and the nearest school that had that option was one hour's travel away. When she was 17, Sophie decided that she wanted to go to Spain for one year, where she completed the equivalent of her 'A-levels'. She stayed with a Spanish family in Madrid and helped look after their children whilst attending school. Although the parents in this host family could speak French, and would occasionally use a French word to help Sophie out, she spoke and heard almost exclusively Spanish and by the end of the year she was totally fluent.

Saadia

However, probably the most remarkable example of interviewees making their own decisions about languages is Saadia, who was being raised primarily bilingually in Punjabi and English but decided when she was around 11 that she wanted to start speaking Urdu. (Saadia had had the opportunity to attend Urdu Saturday school for a couple of years when she was around six or seven). Saadia's family have relatives in both Pakistan and India. When Saadia was about 10 years old, a series of relatives came over to live with them including her brother's new wife, her sister-in-law. Some of these relatives spoke Urdu but no Punjabi. Saadia's parents switched into speaking Urdu when these visitors were living with them, especially at the beginning of the visits, although the visitors also picked up Punjabi so that the language pattern started to become very mixed. Saadia saw this as an opportunity to learn Urdu. She developed a passionate interest in the Urdu language, for reasons that she cannot fully explain. 'I was speaking so much Punjabi …just without thinking and I was paying a lot of attention to my Urdu because I wanted to speak fluently with my sister-in-law. She used to read lots of magazines, books and I was just in awe … the words were so elaborate and long and so many things that I had not heard before. So by the time I was 16, I was probably speaking Urdu better than Punjabi, because I had this passion…'. She remembers on a visit seeing two cousins who had gone to Urdu school doing some work out of books in Urdu and she remembers being jealous of them and at that point wishing that she had kept going to Urdu school.

Another way in which interviewees asserted control, more negatively, over their linguistic upbringing was to resist speaking a parent's preferred language. A whole section of this book is devoted to the issue of resistance as it is so common, and as it causes so much concern to Waltham Forest Bilingual Group members and parents who have attended our workshops (see Chapter 11, p.81).

Conclusion

- The above examples are a salutary reminder that children are most definitely not passive containers waiting to be filled with whatever languages their parents have the desire and capacity to give them, but actively decide what they prefer to speak both on a day-to-day and long-term basis.
- This means that you need to try to create a situation whereby a child positively *wishes* to speak a language.
- As with Saadia, this could be because they associate the language with someone that they admire.
- It could also be because they have had a lot of fun and positive experiences in that language.
- Children also respond well when they want to communicate with monolingual speakers that they care about in that language.

PART 2

Issues at Home that will Affect Most, if Not All, Families at Some Time

9 Consistency Versus Flexibility in Languages Used at Home

10 Rewards, Encouragement, Sanctions and Disapproval Linked to Language Use

11 Resistance – Children Who Prefer Not to Speak a Language

12 Fitting In/Standing Out

13 Input from Others, Resources and Holidays

In this part of the book I discuss many issues that are of concern to most, if not all families at some point or another. One common concern is whether it is best to have a set of consistent rules and strictly (try to) make sure everyone follows them, or to have a more flexible approach. I cover what interviewees' parents did to reward and encourage their children to speak particular languages and whether any sanctions were applied or disapproval voiced if they did not do so. I also set out five examples of interviewees who consistently did not speak the language their parents would have preferred, and I show how this was either overcome by the family or changed when the child became a young adult. Finally, in this section, I analyse what interviewees said that they felt as children about fitting in/or standing out, being different. Some were positive and proud to be different, whereas others had short-term concerns at times, although these were not deeply felt. Only two felt really strongly that they would have preferred it if they could have avoided having to be 'different'.

9 Consistency Versus Flexibility in Languages Used at Home

One of the common pieces of advice in books about bilingualism is that multilingual families should try to establish a consistent set of rules regarding when, where or by whom different languages are used. The advice usually goes on to say something along the lines that there is no right or wrong point or way to fix the boundaries; it is more important to have rules and to stick to them than the particular set of rules you pick. This is something that parents very often ask about at WFBG workshops. Some parents find it difficult to stick to any rules and worry that if they do not manage to do so this will impact on their children's language development. Others picked a system before they knew very much about raising children bilingually and now want to change it, but worry that this will confuse the children. Still more have chosen systems that seemed to give the children the best balance between languages at the time, but want to change this because their circumstances have changed. Finally, parents find it very hard to find a balance between being overly strict (causing a backlash) or overly lax (resulting in a language getting lost entirely). Some parents worry that, if they try to maintain a very strict system, the children will resent this and that this will affect their relationship and/or turn them off the language entirely – and stories about children who have reacted in this way do the rounds and give parents sleepless nights. Other parents worry that if they are not strict enough the children will just stop speaking a language because of peer group pressure and wanting to fit in.

As this is such a common issue for parents, we asked interviewees about this. Some remembered the family having strict rules, others had established language habits that never needed to be enforced, and some recalled that there were no rules. In our interviewees' families we found 'one person, one language' rules, and 'one place, one language' rules. Several families had evolved a rough system whereby different subjects or types of conversation tended to take place in different languages. 'One time, one language' rules did not seem to be very successful. We also found many different variations and combinations and, of course, in some families patterns changed over time.

When discussing this, several questions arise – What systems did families have? What range of factors were language use rules linked to? Were the rules strict or flexible? Or more to the point, who did, and who did not, follow the rules? There was a lot of variation in this whole area within our sample of interviewees. Some families did have rules and kept to them. Some started out with rules but became more flexible. Others had flexibility in certain areas, whilst yet more had a very great deal of flexibility indeed.

I will start with the families that were most consistent, before moving on to those who were more flexible or where patterns changed over time, and finishing up with those who were very flexible – some to the point that they had no rules at all.

Families with Consistent Rules

Saad

There were a number of families that separated languages clearly. Probably the most explicitly discussed example of a family with a very consistent system of language use is that of Saad, who was a Kurdish child, mainly growing up in Arabic speaking Baghdad. Saad was born in Kirkuk, a mainly Kurdish area of Iraq, to a Kurdish mother and father, but the family moved to Baghdad when he was around five. His mother spoke primarily Kurdish but his father was fluent in both Kurdish and Arabic. He has six brothers and sisters, and he is the youngest. The rule in this family was essentially that everyone spoke Kurdish to all the members of his immediate family whether they were at home or outside the house. The whole family spoke exclusively Kurdish at home. Even though Saad's older brothers and sisters learnt Arabic at school, and Saad's father is a fluent Arabic speaker, they *never* spoke Arabic at home. Saad's siblings went to the same school and if they saw each other in the playground they would still speak Kurdish to each other, even though normally at school they spoke only Arabic. The family never used Arabic at home unless they had visitors who could not speak Kurdish. The only exception to this was when Saad's father, who was a devout Muslim, taught his children to recite the Koran in Arabic. Otherwise the only language used in the house was Kurdish. Saad never remembers speaking Arabic at home to his immediate family, not even when discussing something that had come up at school in Arabic. When asked if he knows why this was, Saad says: *'I would say it is something psychological or something natural. ... I cannot speak to them in another language. It would not be real. There was no reason to speak another language to them. If I spoke to them in another language, I would not be myself'*. The family listened to the radio in Arabic, there was TV in Arabic and newspapers in Arabic, but any discussion about the news or content of these media was in Kurdish. *'My parents always said "We are Kurdish and we speak Kurdish in the house".'* Saad's case is interesting because the expectation that he speak Kurdish both at home and outside the home when speaking with another family member seems to have been so strong that he never questioned it. (And this is in the context of hostility between Arabic and Kurdish speakers in Baghdad at this point in time, so speaking Kurdish outside the home would have put the family at some risk of criticism or worse.)

Sylvia

Another example of strict rules was that of Sylvia who grew up the child of two English-speaking parents in France. Sylvia's parents always spoke to her in English. This was a very consistent rule throughout her whole childhood. The family would use

French places and names but otherwise there was very little switching, although Sylvia did hear her parents speak French in their interactions outside the home and so was aware that they were both competent speakers of the language. If Sylvia and her sister met up during break times at school they would speak to each other in English because this is what they did at home.

It seems from our interviews that if and when these sorts of rules begin to slip, this is usually first in conversations between the children. Where this happens, some parents intervene. So in Sylvia's case, she and her sister did bring some French home from school when they played games in French at home that they had learnt from other children in the playground at school. Her mother told them off for speaking French at home, and Sylivia recalls that it was natural for them to comply and switch back to speaking English. She does not remember resisting or resenting this. It seems that Sylvia's mother did not feel that she needed to provide any particular justification for this rule. Interestingly, in Sylvia's case, this relatively strict system seems to have been adopted specifically to benefit the children, as more recently Sylvia has noticed that her parents do mix French and English and speak a lot of 'Franglais'. She feels that her parents have been able to relax their very strict rules about speaking only English now their children have long grown up and left home.

Josune

Josune was the only interviewee in our sample who as a child resented the strict rules that her mother imposed about speaking only Basque at home. Both of Josune's parents were very strict with the use of Basque at home, although her mother was more vocal in her disapproval. *'You could not speak other than in Basque. She would tell us off for speaking in Spanish. She would get very annoyed'*. The only time when Josune's family would allow Spanish to be spoken in the house was when they had visitors who did not speak Basque. As Josune got older she brought home the Spanish that she was increasingly speaking with her friends outside of lessons at her Basque-medium school. When she became a teenager Josune would use an occasional Spanish word with her sisters at home. *'My mother would not like that at all. It had to be purely Basque. She is still like that!'* When she went to a Spanish-medium university, Josune became more influenced by Spanish. *'Occasionally, when I came back home, she would find me speaking Spanish to her. She didn't like that at all. She told me not to speak to her in Spanish ever'*. As a child/teenager, Josune found this attitude very annoying and it made her angry.

Today Josune understands why her parents had this attitude: *'[Basque] was a language that needed support and you needed to look after it, but a teenager does not see it that way. In a way we do have a responsibility of keeping our language, but at the end of it there is a limit, how far you take it within the family …'*. As a result of this experience Josune does not want to impose similar rules on her own children who are growing up with English, Czech and Basque. *'I never want to tell them off for using one language over the other'*.

Saad's father and both Sylvia's and Josune's parents all spoke the majority language well, but in some cases, when insisting that their children speak a certain language at home, the parents pointed out that they did not understand the language spoken in the community. Thus they had a very strong rationale for insisting that at least the conversations between the children and the parents were in one language.

Vera W

Vera W grew up in the UK, the child of two Cantonese-speaking Chinese parents. Both her parents spoke very limited English before they reached the UK, both learnt English whilst here, but both were always much more comfortable speaking Cantonese. Both her parents spoke exclusively in Cantonese to their children. They would get angry with their children if they did not follow their instructions. *'My mother was very upset when we came home from school and we started replying to her in English. She would get cross. She would then say, "In my house, you speak Cantonese, otherwise we won't understand you. Outside the house you speak English, that's fine but here you speak Cantonese. If a relative speaks to you in Cantonese I expect you to reply in Cantonese". She made it very clear that she didn't want us to lose that. We respected that and that is probably why I can still speak Cantonese'.* Although the children respected this rule, there were still some rebellions or some slip-ups. Vera remembers her father shouting at them in Cantonese because they had replied to him in English. She remembers incentives – New Year money – and praise from relatives who noted how good the children's Cantonese was, and how they spoke without an accent.

In this family, the children did speak English together – but only when their parents were not present. Vera would talk Cantonese with her sisters and brother in front of her parents, but they would talk in English when their parents were not around. She remembers that her games were in English: *'All my toys spoke English to each other'.*

Mohammed

Other parents referred to their limited understanding of a language to try to stop their children speaking it, even though our interviewees could clearly see (perhaps in retrospect) that understanding was not, in fact, the issue. Mohammed gave us one example of this. He was raised in the UK speaking Bengali and Sylheti at home and he learnt English at school. From the age of about six to eight or nine, Mohammed and his brothers went through a phase of refusing to speak Bengali/Sylheti at home. He thinks this was because of being at an English school and wanting to fit in. When he did this, his mother would pretend not to understand and would ask him to say whatever he had said again in Bengali/Sylheti. He recalls occasions when it was clear from her response that she had, in fact, understood his question in English:

Mohammed [in English]: *'Mum, can I get 30p for a portion of chips?'*
Mum [in Bengali/Sylheti]: *'Ask me in Bengali and I will give you the money'.*

Like some others, Mohammed noticed that his mother's command of English improved a lot when her children grew up, and he suspects that her refusal to answer

English questions when the children were younger was more as part of a strategy to keep them speaking Bengali/Sylheti than because she did not actually understand them. However, he does also remember some times during this period when his mother genuinely did not understand what one of her sons was saying in English, but his elder sisters would intervene and translate for her.

Saadia

In other cases, the parents' limited knowledge of the majority language was the sole reason why the children did not respond in that language. So although in Saadia's family (Punjabi/Urdu speaking in the UK) there was no rule at all about not speaking English, the children replied to their parents in Punjabi almost all the time while they were at home. If they answered in English, this was acceptable and it was only really the fact that their parents (particularly Saadia's mother) did not speak good English that kept the children speaking Punjabi. Of course though, this pragmatic rationale did not apply to conversations between children, and so in Saadia's family the children spoke English amongst themselves. Despite the fact that Saadia's mother would not have been able to understand all of the details of the conversation between her children in English, Saadia's mother never objected to the children speaking English between themselves in front of her, probably because Saadia's parents felt that it was important that their children speak very good English to do well in life in England.

Antony

In contrast, other parents did mind when conversations between their children were in a language that they did not understand, and so tried to intervene to switch the language between the children back into a preferred language, but unlike Sylvia or Vera W above, this was not successful. Antony's parents moved to England from Cyprus in the 1950s. Both his parents spoke only Greek, although Antony's father could understand and speak some English but not fluently. His parents spoke Greek to each other and to their children, and Antony spoke Greek to them. Antony started to speak much more English when he went to primary school. At this point, he and his sisters all started to speak English amongst themselves. At times when these conversations in English were going on between the children at home, Antony's father became frustrated because he could only understand part of the conversation. Antony's father asked his children to talk to each other in Greek, but the children continued to speak in English. Antony thinks that by this time it was natural for the children to speak in English, and it seems to have become an established habit that was difficult to change. (The fact that their mother could understand none of these conversations did not seem to worry anyone in the family.)

Mumtaz

In another example, this time of a family in difficult circumstances, Mumtaz's mother who spoke Urdu became severely depressed and then mentally unwell when her very young baby died in hospital. Mumtaz was the eldest daughter and assumed a lot of responsibility for her younger brothers and sisters. Mumtaz would normally speak English to them. She did this partly because her mother got upset easily and if she overheard the children talking and understood their conversation, something might set her off. However, on the other hand, her mother would sometimes protest when the children spoke in English: 'She would say "Stop this. Stop this natter-tatter. I don't understand it". And either my sisters and brothers would start to speak to me in their broken Urdu/Punjabi, or I would just break off from what we had been saying and go off and talk to my Mum in Urdu/Punjabi'. Mumtaz's father who spoke English much better than his wife, although not fluently, was working nights and would sleep during the day, and so was not able to spend a lot of time with the family. If he could see that the children were upsetting their mother by speaking English he would ask them to speak in Urdu. However: 'Otherwise, if he walked by as we were speaking [English] he would smile, he was quite pleased'.

You may have noted that none of the examples provided above concern mixed-language families. In our group, although some mixed-language families had strict rules about in which language the parents spoke to the children, almost universally (at least after a certain point) both parents would accept answers from children in either language. Possibly in these families the fact that there are already two languages being spoken within the family makes establishing clear rules more difficult and/or makes any rule harder to stick to.

Mixed-language families typically started out with a strict 'one person, one language' rule (which operated both ways, i.e. not only that the parent spoke to the child in one language but expected a reply in that language too). However, over time, children were gradually allowed to respond to one parent in both languages or even solely in their preferred language, at least about some topics. Interviewees starting school and finding it difficult to discuss what they had learnt in a home language often marked the starting point of a gradual transition away from the strict 'one person, one language' rule operating in both directions. So in Sarah's case of a German/English mixed-language family in Switzerland, although she attended a German-medium primary school for one year, her parents decided to move her to an English-medium school. However, this transition from a German school to an English one eventually affected the language she used when responding to her (German-speaking) mother. She became more proficient in English and less proficient in German. Sarah recalls that it was at this point that she and her brother started to answer to their mother in English, especially when discussing school topics. Sarah remembers that whenever they would sit down to do their homework her mother would ask in German: '"What did you learn today?"' She and her brother would try to explain in German, and then they would switch into English, which became a habit over time. Her mother continued to speak to them in German, and tried to help them with their homework in German as much as she could, but would switch into English at times. This language arrangement was only reserved for school topics and everything else was in German – shopping lists were always in German! However, Sarah also reported that her mother never corrected them if they spoke in English instead of German or asked them to speak to her in a different language.

Shadi (with two Farsi-speaking parents then living in the UK) describes a similar pattern: although her parents spoke mostly Farsi to her, Shadi would reply in a mixture of Farsi and English. For everyday matters she would use Farsi, but to talk about experiences that she had had in English, she would switch into English. *'I would come home from school and I would want to tell my Mum what had happened during the day. I would say in Farsi "And the teacher said ..." and then I would say the rest in English. And my mother would say "Try to say it in Farsi". But I didn't, so whatever I said about school would be in English, although other everyday things would be in Farsi".* In another part of the interview she mentioned that her parents, *'would allow my brother and I to play in English, but when we spoke to them, we were supposed to speak in Farsi'.* She also says that if her father had something particularly serious or important to tell her, he would say it first in Farsi and then would repeat it in English.

More Flexible Rules about Who Speaks What Language at Home

In other families, the position was very flexible with all family members speaking different languages at different times. In Parvati's household in the UK, her mother spoke a mixture of Hindi and English to the children, but her father spoke almost exclusively in English to everyone. Parvati and her sister spoke English to their father and a mixture of both languages to their mother. Thinking about when her mother used which language, Parvati remembers that her mother often used Hindi to discipline the girls: *'She was very articulate in English but when she wanted to order us about she would always speak in Hindi ... When she wanted to get us out of bed or to tell us we had done something wrong, she would use Hindi phrases that there just aren't equivalents for in English. ... I've never thought of it before but the love and the praise was in English, she was a very loving and emotionally connected woman, but that was always expressed in English'.* Parvati did notice some consequences of the fact that the Hindi in her household was alternated with English. She noticed when the family had monolingual Hindi speakers as visitors or nannies that she had to make an effort to not use English words in Hindi sentences.

While Bindi was growing up in Mombasa (the child of third generation immigrants, both Gujarati speakers whose grandparents had migrated from India), the family spoke mostly Gujarati at home, with some English words occasionally interspersed in Gujarati sentences. The family had no TV but they would listen to the radio, sometimes in English, and sometimes in Hindi, and if a comment was made by a family member about what had been said on the radio in English, this might include English words. Visitors would also come from England or Europe, and they would include an English word in a Gujarati sentence.

However, when she was 11 the family moved from Kenya to the UK. Here, they all initially continued to speak Gujarati at home. They had a television for the first time and this brought English into the home. Bindi was aware that her accent in English changed from Kenyan English to North London English and *'I don't remember specific instances, but I can see that there was a stronger influence of English at home than there had ever been before. ... I was using more English than I ever had in Kenya; it was more of a mix'*. Bindi started to reply more often to her parents in English. When Bindi started to speak more English she did not notice a particular reaction from her parents, and she feels that there was an emphasis on the children speaking, reading and writing very good English so as to be able to excel in life as adults. Two years later, Bindi's father was offered work abroad and she and her sister lived with her uncle and aunt (also in the UK). Here *'everyday conversations were in Gujarati, what we were going to eat, what we were going to do, who was coming or going or whatever, but other things were talked about in English, whether it was TV related or the news. We would have a sentence in English and a sentence in Gujarati in the same conversation and it would go backwards and forwards'*.

Other interviewees also recalled that some topics were more likely to be discussed in one language. Later in her interview, Sarah (who, as was discussed earlier, switched from German to English to talk about what had happened at school) described the reverse situation when she mentioned that she speaks better German than her brother, and she thinks this is because she used to talk more about personal things to her mother. *'The fact that I was sharing more personal things with her meant that I spoke German more often'*. When her mother wanted to talk about her feelings, or *'matters of the heart'*, she was much more comfortable speaking in German than in English.

Some interviewees spoke different languages at different periods of their life in response to changes in their parent's preference, and as the parent switched languages the child duly followed this lead. Rose's mother switched the language that she spoke to Rose over time – following shifts in Singapore's national language policies. Initially she spoke Cantonese, but then changed this to Mandarin and finally changed to English, despite the fact that this was *'as she was trying to learn the language herself'*. Rose said that since she was so used to either language it was very easy for her to switch from one to the next, and therefore she always answered in the language her mother spoke to her. She felt very confident in switching between languages as she was raised in a multicultural society where many of her peers spoke different languages.

We mentioned Christine earlier because her German mother who was living in France and who was married to a French man was advised to stop speaking German to her children when Christine was around six years old (for more on this, see page 57 above). Christine does recall that, at some point later, there were some attempts to have days when the family would speak only German, but Christine's brother was unable or reluctant to participate in these and they never really worked.

In Ingrid's case (growing up in Sweden with a Swedish father and an English mother), her mother spoke to Ingrid consistently in English, even though Ingrid replied to her only in Swedish. Ingrid remains grateful that her mother did not insist on her speaking English, and acknowledges that it must have been difficult for her mother to have remained as relaxed about this as she did (see also the more detailed description of this in Chapter 11 on resistance, page 81).

Families With Few or No Rules

Markus

Markus's family were an extreme example of flexibility. Both his parents were linguists and spoke English and German fluently. The language they used to speak to each other was usually English. Both parents spoke both languages to the children, with the aim of achieving a roughly equal balance between English and German. The parents deliberately mixed the two languages and purposely avoided any language boundaries. For example, they would deliberately switch languages mid-sentence ('*Can you please take the Mülleimer out?*'). Markus's family moved between Germany and the United States five times during his childhood. The balance of the languages spoken within the family shifted at these times so that the family spoke more of whichever was not the majority language. These language shifts were a result of the fact that Markus's parents at times noticed that their children's fluency in one language was becoming weaker and they would shift more of their speech into that language. Markus recalls that when he was about six years old and at that time living in the United States, he hardly spoke any German, since he was going to an English-speaking preschool and his German had therefore become '*very weak*'. His parents then decided to speak more German with him in order to redress the balance in his exposure to the two languages. They used the same method later when the family moved back to Germany, when the family language was mainly English. Markus remembers that once the children were a little older (i.e. certainly by the time Markus was a teenager), this switching between sentences no longer occurred, perhaps because the family were living in Germany at this time, and Markus was studying in German and German had become his strongest language so his family had switched to speaking more English at home. In fact, when he was young, language was so natural and not discussed as an issue that Markus could not remember which language he would be using from day-to-day. Only when relatives came to stay or the family moved between countries did Markus again become aware of using any particular language.

Claudia

Claudia, who was brought up in another German/English family, also recalls a similar experience: all of the family switched in and out of their two languages a lot. '*You know starting a sentence in English and finishing it in German … In my case, I never felt it was forced. It was just natural. There was no strict rule, they didn't correct me*'. There was one period which was to some degree an exception to this: '*I think my father at some points got worried because he thought my German was slipping, especially because I was at a German school. So when I started going to German schools in England and Cairo, he spoke German to me a lot because I was in a German education system and had to get my German to a **perfect** level*'.

I described earlier (see p.56) the shift in Sabina's household from Urdu to English when Sabina's mother died, which was only reversed when Sabina's father married her second mother who spoke Urdu but not English.

In Matilde's case, although she reports that her parents spoke only Italian to her and she Italian to them while the family was living in Zaire, in fact some switching of languages had crept in unacknowledged. This became apparent when the family moved back to Italy. Although her family mainly spoke Italian, they did mix French and Swahili words into sentences. When Matilde got back to Italy this was a problem as she found it difficult to say a whole sentence without using French or Swahili words and her friends noticed this.

Two interviewees whose families did allow mixing felt that this had contributed to them either partially losing a language or affected how much of the language they speak today. These interviewees were Sophie, who grew up in south-west France, and Pedro, who grew up in Texas in the United States. Both were in situations where the minority language was stigmatised and low status. It is significant that as both also grew up in bilingual societies, there was no group of people or a place where speaking the minority language was essential in order to be understood. Growing up in a bilingual Spanish/English community, Pedro had to learn to speak English at school without mixing, but (despite the efforts of his father) was more used to mixing English and Spanish languages at home. As all the Spanish speakers in the area also spoke English, there was not an equivalent place where mixing an English word into a Spanish sentence would be unacceptable or where he would not be understood.

Conclusion

Whether families had rules or not, all but one family ultimately succeeded in raising multilingual children speaking the languages that they had hoped for. Only one interviewee (Josune) described resenting her mother's strict rules about speaking Basque at home as a child, although this did not stop her from going to some lengths to speak a minority language (Basque) to her own children, albeit with a great deal of flexibility about who speaks what language. In most families with strict language divisions, the children experienced these rules as natural, and often did not question them. Equally successful in raising bilingual adults were the interviewees who had some rules but were more relaxed about them. Interviewees whose parents switched the language they spoke to them midway through their childhoods were also successful.

A common trigger for the breaking of established rules occurred when interviewees came home from school and wanted to describe their day (and only felt able to do so in the language used at school). Some parents allowed this, and it became normal to talk about school in the majority language with other topics discussed in the minority language. Other families resisted this and conversations about school topics all happened in the minority language. (See Chapter 17, 'Help with Homework', p.139.) Conversations between siblings were also a challenge to many households with rules along the lines of 'we speak x language in this house'. Again, in some families the children were allowed to talk amongst themselves in the majority language (in some cases only when not in the presence of the parents). In some families parents prevented this switch. In one family a father tried to prevent this switch but failed. This may well have been because he raised it too late after the children had established the habit of speaking the majority language to each other both in front of their parents and when on their own.

Interviewees whose parents freely mixed languages were also successful in raising children bilingually. In many cases, these interviewees also functioned in environments outside the home in both languages where mixing was not acceptable (e.g. Markus mixed German and English at home, but at different times attended both English and German-medium schools where mixing the two languages was not acceptable). Parvati very usefully describes how having monolingual Hindi-speaking carers and visitors forced her to stop mixing English into Hindi sentences and to raise her Hindi to a new level (see also p.100).

Sophie was probably the clearest example where flexibility and mixing gradually transitioned into all members of the family speaking the majority language more and more of the time, to the point where Sophie no longer felt able to actively speak Occitan. This shows us that flexibility is only appropriate as long as the overall input of both/all languages is maintained for the children.

Pedro was the second example of a child who grew up with quite a lot of mixing at home, where, in the case of one of his languages, there was not an environment where he needed to speak that language without mixing. Pedro would recommend that parents should not mix languages, if possible, saying that it is easy to mix them if you speak separate languages, whereas it can be hard to separate them if you are used to mixing them a lot of the time. However, if you find it very difficult to stop mixing languages, provided that you maintain the levels of input in both (or more) languages, this may not be a problem if there is another environment where your child needs to speak both of their languages without mixing in order to be understood or to be accepted. This could be a Saturday school or regular holidays in a place whether that language is the majority language.

How you relate to your children is a very personal topic and different people have different styles and approaches, so it is very difficult to give very many pointers in this area. Children also have very different personalities and some may be more willing to accept direction or suggestions from parents (contrast Josune and Rose). So, here is some guidance for you to mull over to work out what is right for you (or use to find a new and different solution for your family).

- Having a system is a good idea, especially when the children are very young – say less than three years old. Children need to learn how to separate their languages, and it helps them do this if their carers at least speak one language at a time. After this, having a system can be useful to ensure that one language does not slip out of the picture almost by accident. Where all the pressures are in one direction, this can happen very easily, gradually, and almost invisibly until you wake up one day and realise that it is too late. Having some sort of system that you more or less stick to guards against this.

- It is relatively easy to have and to stick to a system regarding the languages parents speak to the children, whereas it is much harder to stick to any system when it comes to the languages that children use to reply.
- It is normal for all bilinguals to mix languages when they are speaking to people who speak both languages. Everyone understands and the speech is usually fluent and contains lots of cultural reference points – where the word in the other language is simply not as good. But periodically (after the age of around four or five) you should try to make sure that your children are able to produce sentences in their languages without mixing when they need to (i.e. when speaking to a monolingual speaker of the language). If they cannot do this, try to get them to spend more time interacting with monolingual speakers of that language or put them in settings where mixing is not acceptable (e.g. Saturday school) or visit a place where that language is the majority language.
- If you cannot avoid mixing it is not the end of the world, and there is no need to give up any attempt to raise children bilingually because of this. But do try to arrange for your children to spend significant time with monolingual speakers, or in a setting where mixing will either not get the message across or will not be acceptable.
- Ultimately, it is essential that the children continue to get a reasonable amount of input in each language. If your family might need to move to a new country, you might want or need to change the languages spoken to recreate a good balance (as Markus's family did). In this scenario, it is probably easier to make changes if a relatively relaxed system has been in place until the point when you need to make a switch. If you have had a very strict 'one language at home' policy until this point, then switching this may be more difficult for all involved.
- If you do decide to go for a strict system and your children seem to show signs of resenting this, try to explain to them how important this language is to you. If they are a bit older (probably older than eight years old) see if you can introduce them to a young adult who has lost a language through not speaking it and who now regrets it. Alternatively, try to arrange for your child to have as many fun experiences as possible in that language. Remember that although she resented it at the time and although she does not have any strict rules with her own children, Josune now understands why her mother insisted on her speaking Basque.
- If you have had a fairly strict system, be prepared to defend it when your children start nursery and school, as they are likely to bring the majority language home from school and they may well want to speak it to you as well as to brothers and sisters.
- If you do not want your children to speak a majority language between themselves at home, make this very clear to them from the outset. Once they have a language habit established, it will be very difficult to change. (Even then you may not be able to influence what they speak when you are not there, nor what language they role play in with their toys.)

- Some parents have pretended that they understand less of a language than they actually do in an attempt to keep children speaking a different minority language to them. This can work, unless, of course, in reality, you are a competent speaker.
- If you have a strict system, be prepared for when monolingual visitors are around. Clearly when speaking directly to the visitor(s) you will need to use a language that they understand. But should this mean that you speak exclusively in that language throughout the visit? Some find it very hard to continue to speak a language when there are people in the room who cannot understand it, even when the conversation is not directed at those people. They would say that it seems rude. Others just carry on blithely, happily talking to the children about a problem or an issue in one language and to a monolingual adult in another language (and perhaps translating anything particularly interesting or noteworthy or funny). Clearly if a visitor is a relative who has come to stay for some time, this is more of a problem than if it is a friend coming in for coffee. Just be sure that if you establish one rule for short visits that you do not automatically apply it for long ones. Of course, you can have one practice for when visitors speaking your children's weaker languages come, and a totally different rule for visitors speaking your children's stronger language. (Some people even say that it feels rude to speak a minority language to the children at the supermarket, but I do feel that this is going too far.) It is probably best to start with a system that is very balanced or which is slightly in favour of one or more minority languages – particularly if these are languages that the children do not use at school – as the social pressures will push in the opposite direction over time.
- Remember that children will often accept almost any rule or habit or practice as natural or 'just the way things are'. Even if it feels a bit artificial to you, provided that you start as you mean to go on and proceed with confidence, it will not feel artificial to them.
- If you do evolve a system of speaking two (or more) languages to your children, and tend to use different languages for different topics or subject areas, consider whether you want to use one language or both for certain emotive topics. Using one language to discipline a child, and another language to praise a child, may lead that child to associate negative emotions with the first language and more positive ones with the second. Although Parvati describes this language use pattern (discipline in Hindi, love and praise in English), she does not seem to have formed these emotional associations for the two languages, perhaps because there were many other positive interactions in Hindi (for example, her mother used to sing her children to sleep each night with Hindi songs).

If you are particularly concerned about whether or to what extent you should steer, push or insist with your children about learning a language, you may also want to read the sections covering learning to read and write (starting from p.133). This is because almost all the interviewees who had not learnt to read and write wished that their parents *had* insisted on this or wished that their parents had pushed or encouraged them more.

10 Rewards, Encouragement, Sanctions and Disapproval Linked to Language Use

In this chapter, I discuss parents' methods of encouraging, insisting on or rewarding their preferred language use in particular situations. Again this is an area of very personal choices for parents with many different approaches (including the approach of doing nothing), which can all work very well. One surprising feature of the interviews was the number of cases where interviewees recalled that the language system or choice of language was never an issue, was never discussed and was often treated as a 'given'. In Claudia's case, the tone of her bilingual childhood was that everything was left very natural, nothing was forced, there were almost never any discussions about language or points made about what language should be spoken. Similarly, Sabina said that being bilingual was pretty much taken for granted, a fact of life: *'I don't think anybody ever said to us [when we were children] "That's great – you are bilingual". [Bilingualism] just happened. I think that families that come from abroad view it in a different way. That's just their home language and they are trying to preserve their culture, and language is part of that as well as religion and other things. They don't think of bilingualism in terms of it's good for the brain or can help in job prospects; it is just part of their culture and identity'.* Finally, for Christine, being bilingual just seemed normal. *'It was just part of who I was, I didn't question it really'.*

So, many of our interviewees as children had accepted their language situation as *'just the way things are'.* This applied to some but not all of the cases where the family had strict rules (e.g. Saad, see the discussion above), as well as some but not all of the families that had few or no rules. In the middle, somewhat flexible group, the children of migrants where both parents spoke the same language seemed less likely to discuss language use – although some still did. Mixed-language families seemed more likely to have discussions about which languages should be used and to intervene to support one or more languages, although, again, there were exceptions.

Starting with the more low-key interventions, parents would simply supply a word in a language that they knew the child was trying to remember. When Sarah tried to speak German and was lost for a word and used an English word instead, her mother would give her the German word she needed. She would sense that Sarah was searching for it. Sarah also said that she did not remember her mother praising her when she spoke German and her mother did not correct them if Sarah and her brother spoke in English instead of German.

In other families it seems to have been enough that a parent noticed that a child was tending to slip into speaking the community language rather than the home language. Pari's parents consistently spoke Gujarati to their children, with just the addition of a few English words from time to time. Pari also consistently spoke Gujarati back to her parents, partly, at least initially, because she felt that they would not have fully understood if she spoke in English. Her parents might notice and comment if she included too many English words in her Gujarati sentences, but she was neither punished for speaking English nor rewarded for speaking Gujarati.

Some parents linked speaking languages to pocket money and other treats: Shadi knew that her parents liked to hear her speak Farsi, and she received lots of positive feedback from them about her ability to speak all of her languages. On the other hand *If we spoke too much English, they would take away our pocket money'.*

We described above (p.68) how Vera W's parents linked the giving of New Year money to the children's good Cantonese. Vera also recalls her mother admonishing her elder sister and telling her that Vera's Cantonese was better than hers. In Daniela's case, in order to motivate her to learn Italian, her father used to buy her favourite comics in Italian (Asterix and Obelix).

Some interviewees were aware that there was more praise for the language spoken in the community than the minority language, so Saadia commented, *'We always overlooked the Punjabi and Urdu. It was always "Do well in English, do well at school". If we started going to an Urdu class or developing that language or Punjabi, it would always come second and English would be put first. We were instilled with the sense that English is very important and that to do well you had to be well spoken'.* Compared to this stress on speaking good English, she says: *'We didn't give the [Urdu or Punjabi] language much thought because we were just getting on with it … we had so many things to do, people to meet…'.*

Some interviewees remember a moment when they expected praise from their parents for progress in the minority language, but this did not materialise. Antony was the child of two Greek Cypriot parents living in London. Having really struggled with the Greek alphabet, he came back from Greek school one day able to read and he was proud and expected some acknowledgement from his family, but they hardly seemed to have noticed. The fact that he still remembers that he did not get the praise that he expected shows that this moment struck a chord. You cannot attribute an outcome to any one single event, but nonetheless I will just mention that Antony was one of our interviewees who felt the least confident speaking his second language today.

Conclusion

Rewards and sanctions are a very personal decision for a family. There are really two approaches here. One is to treat the various languages spoken as totally natural, inevitable and 'just how things are'. If you are adopting this approach, you will probably not draw attention to when children speak languages particularly well or choose not to speak a language that you would prefer. The other approach is to discuss the language choices and habits, make a point of noticing things and then you might want to praise and/or reward children and otherwise encourage them in a particular direction. (Within a family, you may have one parent who prefers the first option and one who prefers the second; this is likely to be the case across a wide range of fronts, not just language, and the children will surely cope with it, just as they manage everything else.)

The pointers below are for those taking the second approach:

- Simply noticing and commenting when children use a good phrase or read something in their weaker language may be more valuable than anything else. Perhaps again this is because it conveys to the children that you care about this language. This sounds pretty obvious – but busy real lives tend to intervene and Antony's story reminds me that missing even one opportunity to do this because you are preoccupied with something else or busy may send a message to a child that they remember for a long time.
- You can link presents and rewards to good use of a language, particularly if the present is linked to a celebration of that culture.
- Some parents did withhold some pocket money at times if they felt that a child was speaking too much of the majority language.

11 Resistance – Children Who Prefer Not to Speak a Language

It is extremely common for children to go through a phase whereby they choose not to speak one of their languages at all. During these phases, the children continue to understand the language but choose to answer (either their parents or everyone) in another language (usually the majority language). In mixed-language families this often occurs when children are very young (i.e. under four) although it can also happen later in childhood in both mixed-language and migrant families. It is almost always of great concern to parents who do not know whether to ignore this as a phase which will pass, or whether this is the first step on a slippery slope that will ultimately lead to the loss of a second language. Parents do not know whether or how to intervene or how to persuade a child to speak a particular language. Even if they are tempted to intervene it is not at all clear what they can effectively do. We know that some parents do take this as a trigger to stop speaking a second language to their child.

As we know that this is a major concern for quite a few parents, this chapter is devoted to those interviewees who described having reacted in this way. We hear not only how this felt to them at the time, but also how the interviewees' parents reacted, whether they attempted to challenge or change this and the children's reactions to any attempts at intervention.

Almost all interviewees had moments when they used a language that was not their parents' preferred language, but these were generally quite brief and the usual rules were re-established fairly swiftly (some have been described above, see, for example, Josune, p.67, or Vera W, p.68). In some other cases, the children did continue to use a language other than that which the parent preferred, but these choices were accepted by the parents and so this does not constitute 'resistance' (e.g. see Daniela, p.49, or Sabina, p.55). There were five cases in our sample where interviewees resisted speaking the language that their parents preferred for months or years. Parents often remained very low-key about the fact that they would have preferred a response in a different language, so the distinctions between the interviewees who felt that they were resisting a parent's wish and those who felt that their parent had accepted the choice are quite subtle. Nonetheless, I feel that this distinction did come across in the interviews.

Of the five interviewees, three were in mixed-language families and two were in migrant families. All of the interviewees who resisted continued to have a good passive knowledge of the language as they heard and understood the conversations directed at them in that language. Although we have heard of this happening, there were no straightforward cases where parents stopped speaking to an interviewee in the minority language because the children stopped replying in that language. (There were some interviewees where this happened, see the section on Daniela, whose father stopped speaking Italian to her after her parents' divorce, p.50, and Sabina, whose father stopped speaking Urdu to her after her mother died, on p.55. Other factors were clearly involved in both these cases, and it was also the case that the parent did not have, at that time, a strong preference about the language that the child spoke in so it was not resistance per se in either case.)

In four out of five cases, the interviewees concerned would still speak the language to others (e.g. grandparents, other relatives and friends during visits and holidays) but would not speak to their parent(s) in that language. In the same number of cases, the interviewees' preference in terms of language was reluctantly tolerated by their parents. In only one case was substantive resistance by an interviewee (and two brothers) overcome by a joint family effort. In all four cases where the resistance was maintained through the teenage years, the interviewee then moved to live in a country where their minority language was the majority language as a young adult (without their family) and this seems to have been a significant factor not only in strengthening their knowledge of this language but, in three of the four cases, prompting the interviewee to switch to start speaking it to their parent again (for more details specifically on this see also Chapter 23 on studying and working abroad as young adults, p.173). As adults all five interviewees in this group have returned to speaking the language that they refused to speak (to their parents) as a child, mostly very enthusiastically, although, in one case, with less confidence. As this issue causes so much concern to parents (and comes up again and again at WFBG workshops), I will describe all five cases in a little detail, starting with the family that managed to overcome the resistance.

Mohammed

Mohammed grew up in London, the child of migrants from Bangladesh who spoke Bengali and the Sylheti dialect of Bengali. Mohammed's father also spoke fluent English. For two to three years, starting when he was around six years old, Mohammed and his brothers tried to refuse to speak Bengali/Sylheti at home. He thinks this was because of being at an English school and wanting to fit in. Mohammed thinks that he (and his brothers) switched back to speaking Bengali/Sylheti when he was eight or nine because his elder sisters and brothers all spoke Bengali/Sylheti, and insisted that all of the children did too.

There were complex and fascinating reasons behind this struggle over language in this family, which Mohammed has reflected on and shared with us very thoughtfully. Mohammed explains that Bengali/Sylheti is a language that involves referring to people who are older than you with respectful titles such as 'aunty' or 'uncle' or (more galling for Mohammed) '[elder] sister' or '[elder] brother'. These terms convey respect but also place the two speakers in a hierarchy. There are also two forms of 'you': one more formal for elders and one less formal - similar to the French 'vous' and 'tu'. Mohammed is the seventh of eight children and his eldest sister is 17 years older than he is. He and the two brothers closest to him in age were reluctant to speak Bengali/Sylheti at home because needing to start a conversation with the phrase 'Elder sister', which automatically conveyed respect and a hierarchical relationship between the speakers, put them at a disadvantage and they tended to lose every argument or discussion – as was expected in Bengali/Sylheti culture. Their elder siblings, however, preferred to speak Bengali/Sylheti for the same reasons (i.e. they tended to win every discussion). *'By the time I was eight years old I knew that English was a more egalitarian language – I knew this because of the way my teachers spoke to me'.*

Ingrid

For many years, Ingrid refused to speak English to her American mother who lived in Sweden. Ingrid started off as a very young child speaking more English than Swedish, but during her first years at school, Ingrid's language preference started to change and she preferred to speak Swedish, and eventually she always answered her mother in Swedish even though her mother very consistently spoke only in English to her. Her mother did not seem worried by this and never put her under pressure to speak English. *'I am very grateful to her for that – that she didn't pressure me into speaking English with her. I know that it must have been difficult'.* The family twice tried to relocate back to the United States from Sweden, once spending six months there during which time Ingrid went to school (she was about nine years old), and once spending four months there during the summer. However, for work reasons, this never worked out and each time they returned to Sweden.

Nonetheless, each summer the family would go for long holidays to the United States to stay with relatives and see a network of Ingrid's mother's close friends. Each year, initially, it was difficult for Ingrid to speak English, but after a few days had passed she found that she could speak English without any problems. By the end of the holidays, when the family returned to Sweden, she would have the same slight problem in switching back to speaking Swedish, although, again, after a few days this would pass. Thus, Ingrid's mother may have been reassured by the fact that she knew her daughter could speak English when she needed to. Ingrid, whose Swedish father died when she was 11 years old, consistently refrained from addressing her mother in English until she was almost grown up. *'It was not until I was 16 and I went to study in the States that I started to speak English back to [my mother]'.* Ingrid now lives in the UK, is married to a Swedish man and is raising her own children bilingually in Swedish and English.

Helen

Helen, the child of an English father and a Dutch mother living in Holland, also preferred to speak Dutch and would not speak English at home from an early age. She says that she was perhaps embarrassed to answer her father in English or felt that there was some barrier that prevented her from replying in English. She also says that it seems that Dutch simply came more easily and quickly to her. She does not remember him responding negatively to this. She was neither punished nor rewarded at home for speaking a particular language. She has been told though that her father was aware of another family where a child had been strongly pushed to use their weaker language (also English) and this had been counterproductive, and the child had developed a complex about speaking English. Hence he preferred to keep things low-key. Helen spoke English with her English relatives and on visits to England, and so her parents were aware that she could speak English when she needed to.

Helen is now studying in the UK and, as a result, she says that her English is getting stronger, although she still feels that Dutch is her first and strongest language. She speaks Dutch to her family when in Holland, and English when in England. She has a Dutch accent when she speaks English, but she also says that people say that she has a slight accent when she speaks Dutch. After we had met and talked, Helen spoke to her father about how he had felt when she refused to reply to him in English. He sent her the following email, which she then kindly sent to our team. When I was analysing all the material for the book, I asked her if I could include part of it because I found it very informative and moving.

Yes, I was sometimes frustrated that you didn't reply in English. It felt a bit like a denial of my (and your) roots. That I had to give way to the prevailing culture even in my communication with my own children. I hope I didn't make that too obvious at the time, but knowing me, I probably did a bit. It came home to me when you moved to England and got married in the town where I was born that it meant much more to me than I'd ever realised it could do. When you started to email me in English it felt as though we had reached a new level of intimacy that we'd not had before. ... I always hoped that you and your brother would embrace both languages and make them your own, in order to have a more varied palette with which to express yourselves. It makes me happy to know that that has happened.

Lots of love,
Papa (not Dad or Daddy, but I'm quite happy and have grown used to being Papa!) xx

Camilla

In Camilla's case, as a very young child, Camilla heard and spoke only Danish at home. When she started nursery aged around two and a half, her parents sought the advice of teachers and were told that they should continue to speak Danish at home and that she would pick up English quickly at school. They followed this advice and Camilla did pick up English quickly. Within a very short time, Camilla was very fluent in English – although being somewhat perfectionist she would point out that she still made occasional mistakes with a saying or odd word. However, not long after starting at nursery, she started to refuse to speak Danish at home. *'I think I didn't want to be different. I remember feeling **so** different, and I didn't want to be ... all through my childhood I felt different. I used to get words for things wrong at school. I used to get my English and Danish* *muddled up. Pancakes I called panacakes (because that's the word in Danish). So I really worked hard to be as English as I could, so I fitted in. I remember other children laughing at me, [when I made mistakes] which I hated'.* Camilla's parents did not seem to worry that she had stopped speaking Danish. She still had a good passive knowledge as she understood all the Danish being spoken to her and around her at home. (Her brother, who is 13 years older than her, had lived in Denmark until he was 11 and spoke Danish to his parents at home.) She does not remember any pressure, any rewards or any punishment linked to which language she used, and her parents seem just to have accepted her decision to speak English. Camilla describes her home life as very relaxed with little pressure from her parents in any area.

Like other interviewees, Camilla spoke Danish when visiting friends and family in Denmark, although, unlike others, she commented: *'I guess that I am particularly shy of speaking Danish in front of my parents although if we go on holiday, I can speak Danish in front of people I don't know much more freely'.* When she was seven, Camilla went to Denmark to visit family and friends and met a lifelong friend, Nanna, who was the same age as her. She remembers that her ability to read and write in Danish was much better than this friend (as school starts much later in Denmark). And she remembers that she had no problems speaking Danish with her grandparents and Nanna and her family. So, at this point, she was still very comfortable speaking Danish despite having stopped speaking Danish to her parents at home several years earlier.

Also, it is interesting that not speaking the language was not linked to any negative feelings about Danish culture. Despite not speaking Danish at home, Camilla still had a very positive attitude towards Denmark and she remembers celebrating Danish festivals, and Danish food. Her toys also had Danish names. When she was 16 she says, *'I wanted to leave school and go and finish my schooling in Denmark. I was really set on that. But my father put his foot down and said that I had to finish my schooling in England. He was an academic, and he wanted to me to go to university in the UK, and I think that it was probably a good decision because I think I would have had a good experience but I would have struggled because I couldn't really write Danish'.*

When she was about 18 years old Camilla went to live in Denmark for three months (staying with her friend, Nanna's family) and worked in the local council, so at this point she was also able to hold down a job in Danish. Looking back today, Camilla did regret that she stopped speaking Danish. *'It's taken me a long time to get to grips with the fact that I left the Danish behind and I felt really guilty And I wish that I hadn't. I sometimes wish that my parents had not let me, had made me speak Danish at home. But then I think that I was unhappy speaking it so ...'*

She also said: *'For years I would just avoid speaking Danish, but now I have decided just to try speaking Danish to everybody when I'm over there. I've enjoyed it a lot more since I gave up my Danish passport. Now I am an English person who can speak Danish, rather than someone who is Danish but who can't speak Danish perfectly'.* Camilla still speaks English to her parents today and she prefers to speak English with her Danish friends who are living in the UK.

Armelle

Our final example of resistance is Armelle and is slightly less clear-cut. Armelle grew up in a mixed language family with a French father and Argentinean mother, and moved between Argentina, France and Italy during her childhood. (She was the only interviewee whose parents had decided to each speak their own language to the other.) Initially, Armelle did reply to her mother only in Spanish when they were speaking one-to-one, but later, when the family had moved first to France and then to Italy (attending French-medium schools throughout), both Armelle and her brother started to also reply to their mother in French, even though she always spoke Spanish to them. Armelle and her brother mixed quite a lot of French and Spanish in conversations with their mother. However, they spoke exclusively in French to their father and also in French between themselves. *'So even when we are eating at the table, three of us speak French and my mother speaks Spanish'.* Armelle's mother never seemed to worry that Armelle would lose her Spanish. She encouraged her children to write to their Argentinean grandparents each week – but this was as much about ensuring that they had a relationship as about maintaining the language.

Every year the family went to Argentina for one month to give the children access to their cultural heritage. This meant that they could meet up with their large family there. Armelle's grandparents would also come to stay with the family in Europe for several months at a time, and would help to care for their grandchildren. Although Armelle's Argentinean grandparents could speak and understand some French, they only ever spoke to them in Spanish. Thus again Armelle's mother knew from these holidays and visits, as well as from some mixing in conversations with her, that her children could still speak as well as understand Spanish. However, the basic pattern of Armelle speaking French to her Spanish-speaking mother persisted for a long time – until Armelle was 24. *'When I was 19 I went to live in Argentina, I went to university and I was in touch with my large Argentinean family, my parents had gone to work elsewhere. When they came back to live in Argentina, and I lived with them again, I started to speak exclusively Spanish to my mother, and after this it felt strange to speak to her in French. It was very strange'.* Thus once again, after a break which involved living in a place where Spanish was the majority language, Armelle finally switched to speaking the language that her mother would have preferred all along.

If you have read all of the book until here and have not dipped in and out, you may recall the discussion about Sophie who grew up speaking French, Occitan, and Spanish as a child and who has also learnt fluent Italian (for more on Sophie's experiences, see p.25). Sophie's case cannot be characterised as resistance because her parents had internalised some of the negative views in sections of their community towards Occitan and so did not encourage Sophie to speak it. However, Sophie did comment on the fact that she finds that she cannot speak Occitan as an adult, and I would like to include a quote here as this may shed some light on how children actually feel when they will not or cannot respond in a parent's preferred language. In Sophie's case, since she is an adult and a clinical psychologist with a well-developed ability for introspection and reflection, the issue is 'cannot' rather than 'will not'. When asked what languages she would speak to any children she may have in the future Sophie says: *'All of them, except Occitan. Because I couldn't pass it on. There's no way for me to pass it on. I wouldn't know where to start [to speak it]. I can hear it in my head, if I need to say something ... but it doesn't come out'.*

Conclusion

If your child prefers not to speak one of their languages to you, this does not mean all is lost. Interviewees who resisted speaking one or both parents' preferred languages all ended up fluent speakers of that language (in one case less confidently).

In all of these cases, one or both parents was a first language speaker of the language and continued to speak it to the child. If you take your child's resistance to mean that you should give up speaking that language to them, they will almost always start to lose that language quite rapidly. In the cases where parents did allow a child's switch to trigger them to also change languages, this led to a rapid deterioration in the child's knowledge of that language. In Daniela's case, her father not only accepted her responses in French and not Italian but answered her in French too, and although Daniela can still speak Italian she feels less confident and that she needs to practise and to develop more mature language in Italian (she is still bilingual in English and French). (For more about Daniela and the impact of her parents' divorce, see p.55). In Sabina's case, she had more or less lost her Urdu in the two years between her mother's death and her father's remarriage to a monolingual Urdu-speaking woman, which meant that she had to rapidly reacquire Urdu. (For all the details of Sabina's story, see p.55.)

In all our five cases at least one parent continued to speak a minority language to the child, and although the interviewees' responses in another language were acceptable to the parent, the child still knew (in some cases only very subtly) that the parent would have preferred the response in another language.

If you have a child who is resisting speaking a particular language and you are not the sort of family where the parents simply insist on something and it is done (see Sylvia, p.66, and Vera W, p.68), this suggests the need for some tightrope walking.

- Do not stop speaking your language to your child. As long as they continue to hear the language, they will continue to understand it. This means that they have a passive knowledge of the language. It is certainly much easier to go from the ability to understand a language to being able to speak it than having to learn it almost from scratch. Four of our interviewees did make this transition with apparent ease.
- Continue to convey (subtly if you prefer) to your child that the language that they are choosing not to speak is very important to you and you would prefer that they speak it.
- You can try to mount a campaign, as Mohammed's family did, to push the children to speak the minority language. Camilla half wishes that her parents had pushed

her more, but also recognises that this would have made her unhappy and so respects their decision. We are not aware of many such campaigns that have been successful, but then perhaps Josune, Vera W or Sylvia would have resisted if strict rules had not already been established. (See the section on families with strict rules from p.66.)

- Be aware that if you do insist or push that your child may ultimately feel resentful or may feel that they need to stick to their guns to make a point.
- If possible arrange visits to a country where the resisted language is the majority language and, if possible, time for your child with monolingual children (or second best, adults). Your child will normally produce speech – especially to other children or to relatives that they care for and are comfortable with – and this is great for them to practise actively speaking. It will also be very reassuring to you to listen in (or bearing in mind Camilla's point about being sensitive to her parents listening to her talking Danish, hear about). Do not be surprised if they continue to speak their usual, non-preferred language to you throughout.
- Do not be surprised if your son or daughter is interested in spending time as a young adult in a context where the resisted language is the majority language. It is possible that doing so may finally trigger a change in the language that they use to speak to you.

Good luck!

12 Fitting In/Standing Out

Interviewees generally became conscious of differences between themselves and their peers, and became aware of what is considered 'normal', during their primary school years. More than half of our interviewees mentioned being aware of being different, and spoke of wanting to fit in at some point or other during their childhoods. Some of the interviewees were being raised bilingually in bilingual cities or countries or were attending bilingual schools and they were, in fact, no different from their peers in terms of language use. For these interviewees, the issue of wanting to fit in (or not) did not arise. For some interviewees in monolingual schools that had a rich mix of pupils, again wanting to fit in was not an issue. One example of this is Christine, for whom being bilingual just seemed normal. In her school outside Paris, there were many other children in her class who spoke other languages at home (mainly European languages – German, English, Danish, Portuguese). Many of these children started school speaking either limited French or no French at all. Christine recalls no disapproval from teachers about this and cites this as one reason why she felt that being bilingual was normal and positive.

Where interviewees did perceive differences between themselves and other children, race, religion and ethnic origin were very often bound up with linguistic differences. These different aspects of identity, or of how we are perceived by others, are very hard to separate out. Almost 30 interviewees were linguistically different from the majority of their peers. Of these, one quarter either did not mention it or explicitly said that (at least in terms of language) this was not an issue for them at all. For example, Sabina – who spoke Urdu at home went to a school in England that was ethnically mixed in terms of white and African/Afro-Caribbean children but had few Asian children – remembers standing out because she wore trousers or because she was Asian, but never because of her ability to speak Urdu. Although Zwelibanzi did mention that he was the only Zulu-speaking boy out of 700 students at his school, he raised no issues linked to this.

Interviewees With Some Concerns

Just over half of our interviewees had had some concerns at some point about wanting to fit in. Many of those who remembered feeling concerned gave examples of small adjustments to their behaviour so as to be able to fit in more or stand out less. In most cases, this concern about fitting in was both minor and transitory, interviewees either resolved it or grew out of it, but in one or two cases it seems to have continued for longer and to have run deeper. Only five interviewees remember seeing their difference as a positive when they were children (although all saw their difference as positive once they were adults).

Matilde was very explicit about being viewed as different although it is atypical that she became aware of this at a relatively late age. When she was 15 and her family returned from Zaire to Italy, she says: *'We were always the weird family. People back in Italy found it strange that my family had lived in Africa. ... It's difficult when you're fifteen. That was the most difficult part. Teenagers have their rules, and I had been used to society in Goma'.* Later she also said, *'I have always been proud of my languages. I always felt as a child that it was something that was admired. It was a plus. But I did find it difficult travelling so much – being seen as weird'.*

This would strike a chord with Sarah who, when people ask her where she is from, tells them that she is not from any place in particular and lists all the places she belongs to. When she says that she speaks three languages, she sometimes feels she should be a little *'apologetic'* about it, and feels like an *'exotic bird'*, and at times feels that people become a bit cautious towards her. As a consequence she feels she needs to downplay it so she is not too different from everybody else.

Mohammed was also conscious of wanting to fit in and went to some lengths to change his accent so that he would do so. As recounted in the previous chapter (p.82), wanting to fit in may have been behind his (failed) attempts to switch the language he spoke back to his parents to English. Interestingly, however, even though Mohammed did not have a Bengali accent when he spoke English, the very correct, formal and old-fashioned English he learned from his father would have made him stand out. He remembers wanting to fit in and he and his brothers consciously adapted their speech – using a London cockney accent, which is how the majority of people on his East London estate and at his school spoke. He remembers that one of the first books he owned when he was eight was a dictionary of cockney rhyming slang, which he read to make sure that he had got his cockney right. He recalls using a cockney accent, cockney phrases and rhyming slang at home but being corrected by his father who told him to speak properly. Mohammed never had any problems with switching between different languages or different dialects of languages, and he thinks that the fact that he had already been taught the difference between the more formal Bengali and the dialect Sylheti helped him to also switch between Cockney at school, and more formal English in the presence of his father.

Bindi also changed her accent. She slightly more ambiguously tells us that her school had perhaps only one or two Asian pupils, with the vast majority of students being white. Despite this, *'I myself have never felt stigmatised ... I kept [the languages] quite separate. I was teased because my English accent was different, but I never spoke Gujarati at school – at school I stuck to English'.* In fact, after the move to London, Bindi was aware that her accent changed from Kenyan-English to North London-English, which may have been in reaction to the fact that she had been teased.

Another interviewee aware of being different was Parvati. She and her sister were the only two ethnic minority children at their primary school. She remembers *'I was always aware that it made us different. I remember when I wrote about what I had done at the weekend, or what we had eaten, I remember feeling uncomfortable ... I would always have a little glossary at the end to explain – this is what a salwa kameese is ...'.* (Fortunately her teacher was positive about these glossaries.)

Vera W was teased at school by other pupils because she was Chinese. *'As I was growing up in school, I was made to feel very different. There was nobody who was Chinese at my school. There were very few other children who spoke a second language at home. I was teased in the playground, racial comments were made and I remember being very upset. My friends told me not to take any notice of them and I remember the teacher making it clear in class that this was not acceptable. I remember being in tears in class because of this'.* By then, Vera spoke English without an accent and these comments were due to her physical appearance (i.e. this was essentially racism). But, she says, *'... for me this was also about language'.* Her first secondary school was more mixed with Japanese and Korean children whose parents had come to work in the UK for one year. There were also children born here who had different backgrounds, spoke a different language at home, and ate different foods (e.g. a Hindi speaking family of Indian origin). *'These children were very aware of the culture they came from and that changed me'.* The family then moved to Oxford, where she went to a fee-paying school; again she was the only Chinese child, but here she found the other children were more tolerant and open: *'They were not brought up to be racially prejudiced. I remember bringing it up in a discussion at school, I said "I **am** different" but they said "No you're not, you speak English, you are English"'.* These children did not see Vera's physical Chinese appearance as at all significant, and they cited her native English as a reason to consider her to be just like them.

We will discuss Marion's difficulties at school in Chapter 14 (see p.111), but it is worth mentioning here that the turning point for her (which turned her from a special needs child to a high achiever) came when Marion was *'in an environment where I wasn't mocked, where I was considered "normal".... There was sufficient bilingualism around to give you a feeling that it was OK. Many teachers were bilingual'.*

Sophie was another child who was conscious of being different where she grew up in south-western France. Linguists consider Occitan a distinct language, but in France it is widely referred to as a degraded version of French. This meant that Sophie felt different from her monolingual French friends, and also from other bilingual children. When Sophie's school friends came to stay or to play, they would notice that her grandparents would speak Occitan, would clearly not understand what was being said, and Sophie would translate so that her friends could follow what was going on. When this happened she says: *'I felt different ... do I fit into this? Even though there were a lot of bilingual children (Dutch and English) whose families had moved into the area. ... I didn't consider myself like them because for me it [French and Occitan] was one language. Remember [Occitan] wasn't considered a language – it was a lesser ... something. It's sad'.* However, Sophie's view did change later. *'As I grew older and I met more foreigners and I started to make connections ... as a teenager I realised that I **was** like those bilingual children that I knew'.*

In Daniela's case, it was her mother who may have wanted to fit in. Daniela's mother had moved back to the UK from Italy after separating from Daniela's Italian-American father. Daniela thinks that keeping up Italian in a new environment was very difficult as she was living with her mother in a *'parochial community'* (on a farm in Hertfordshire in England). This was a *'very close knit, old-fashioned village where people were quite suspicious...you know...this was 1964...of newcomers, and certainly anybody foreign, so the fact that she had this small toddler speaking in a foreign language was a bit strange, and I think she was trying to fit in and maybe didn't want me to stand out too much...'.* This led her mother to stop speaking to her in Italian, which, combined with other factors (see p.50), meant that Daniela lost a lot of her fluency and confidence in speaking Italian.

Those interviewees who spent much or all of their childhoods in international schools surrounded by other multilingual children are interesting in this context, if, for a short part of their childhood, they moved into more traditional national state schools where most or all of their peers were monolingual. This allowed them to contrast situations where they were no different from their peers with situations where they stood out. This happened to (German and English-speaking) Claudia, who attended international schools whilst her father was posted overseas as a diplomat, but went to an ordinary German state school when he was posted home to Germany. In the international schools being multilingual was the norm. *'Everyone I went to school with (except in Germany) spoke at least two languages, many spoke three languages. ... Probably I stuck out most in Germany,... that's when I really stuck out ... it was only there that it was an issue but it was never really a big issue – I was never bullied or picked on or anything'.* Claudia only recalled one other point: *'I remember people saying "You're showing off". Children in Cairo who had just come from Germany [who could speak only German] would say this and say "Stop speaking English", even though most of the class, in fact, spoke English'.* Because of this, Claudia says she does not advertise her bilingualism to all and sundry: *'So it's not something that I necessarily bang on about'.*

Armelle (who speaks Spanish, French and Italian) switched from international schools to a state secondary school in France, where she was the only multilingual child. She felt that the other students admired the fact that she spoke several languages. *'At that moment I realised that I was very lucky. The French exams are very tough to pass, including languages, but for me it was very easy'.* Armelle also felt that she stood out more when she went to university in Argentina, where the teachers were amazed that she was completely bilingual. Generally, Armelle was admired for her knowledge of French language and culture, although less positively she also encountered some jealousy from other students at her university.

Two remaining interviewees seemed to feel the discomfort of not fitting in most acutely. Interestingly, neither of them was racially or religiously different from their peers, and the difference that they struggled with was purely linguistic. Camilla had grown up in the UK speaking Danish at home but, as discussed in the chapter on resistance (see p.84), had stopped replying to her parents in Danish not long after starting school. Camilla was one of very few children in her class who spoke a language other than English at home. She loved the different food they ate, the traditions and festivals that her family celebrated, and she says that her family was very Danish – all her toys had Danish names, and they used Danish-style decorations in the house and at birthday parties. Her close friends admired this and seemed to find her family exotic in a positive way. But, as a young child, she did not like to stand out. She remembers that when she was older (in her late teens) being different was seen as being more positive, but she remembers that younger children can be quite cruel without intending to be. *'I think I didn't want to be different. I remember feeling **so** different, and I didn't want to be … all through my childhood I felt different. I used to get words for things wrong at school. I used to get my English and Danish muddled up. … So I really worked hard to be as English as I could, so I fitted in. … I remember other children laughing at me, [when I made mistakes] which I hated'.* At the end of the interview, she repeats that, *'I think what I most wanted was to just fit in and to speak English'.*

Sylvia grew up the child of English parents living in France. She told us: *'In the summer I was the French girl in England, and the rest of the year round I was the English girl in France'.* At one point in the interview she said she recalled being the only bilingual child in her school, until a German boy also joined the school. She remembers being aware that other families did do things differently and she remembers being 'different' and not always liking that. However, this was as much about culture and the things that families did, as about language per se, and Sylvia also says that she just took the situation and her ability to speak two languages for granted. Later on though, in a reversal of Claudia and Armelle's experience, she could contrast state schools and an international school, but in her case she had spent most of her school life in the state system and she experienced the international school as a distinct relief: *'I did grapple with being French or English without there ever being any specific issue – nothing done in my friends' houses and not in mine that I resented and no big crisis or cultural clash. …[But it] was an enormous relief to join the international lycée and meet other people "like me". I know the sense of not belonging was a sense that many of us in that school had experienced and the sense of belonging within the school was intense because whatever our nationality and languages we all shared that very unique thing of being an outsider (and of being able to speak several languages of course). It was a bond and I am still in touch with friends from that school and know that many more are still in touch with each other'.* Later in the interview she also says: *'Why I haven't focussed on languages for my career is also bound up with the outsider/migrant thing. As any career based on languages would logically require me to travel it would forever perpetuate the business of being an outsider and not belonging anywhere - and of course probably moving on regularly. I wanted to be "normal" and have a normal life that stayed in one place'.* (Sylvia chose to be a lawyer and is successfully practising in a large City of London law firm).

Interviewees Who Viewed Being Different as a Positive

Other interviewees had views that were more mixed. Markus was always happy that he was able to speak two languages and thought it was a good thing to have something that others did not have. It did make him feel different from his peers in that to a certain extent he perhaps felt excluded from them, or he felt that he was not at home in either place. Overall, he saw it as both a negative and a positive thing; although he saw speaking two languages as a special skill and valuable, he also felt at times that *'like you're not fully German nor fully English speaking – always a bit of a stranger in either language. Perhaps you're just more aware of languages in general and so more aware of mistakes you make'.*

At her primary school, Helen's teachers were positive about her bilingualism. When her class started learning basic English in the last two years of school, Helen would often be asked to read out the text to the class. There was another girl in her class who spoke Italian at home and the two of them would almost show off to their peers about the fact that they spoke another language. The teachers were equally positive about the Italian girl's language, so this was not just because many Dutch people speak English and it is the first foreign language taught in school that they were positive about Helen's home language.

Shadi was the child of Iranian parents who fled Iran and who lived in France and the UK before finally settling in Sweden. Shadi learned Swedish very quickly when she moved to Sweden aged 12. She also spoke Farsi, English and French. Shadi was always proud to be able to speak more than one language: *'I would say I was always quite admired for speaking different languages. People would say "Oh you're so lucky". So I gained popularity at school. … I think we were lucky as we were the first Iranians to come to this town in northern Sweden and we were very exotic … we were interviewed on the radio. I remember that four years later, when a lot of Iranians had come, it wasn't that popular anymore and Iranian children were bullied in school because they couldn't speak Swedish'.*

Ingrid, also in Sweden, told us that her mother was the only non-Swedish person in her village and this did make the family stand out. This was a positive thing as her mother was American, but Ingrid wonders if people would have been less positive if her mother had been from Asia or Africa.

In Saad's case, being Kurdish and being different was about a lot more than perception and 'fitting in'. In Baghdad there was a lot of racism against the Kurds. At this time, there was a war going on between the Iraqi government and the Kurdish rebels. The situation was very political and very tense. There was a lot of nationalism. Many people in Iraq hated the Kurds and this was especially true in the area Saad lived in. Despite this difficult situation, the family did not try to hide their Kurdishness and Saad would never deny his origins.

Saadia was the interviewee who actively went out of her way to be different in terms of her language choices. She describes herself when very young as a very shy child, which other interviewees have associated with not wanting to be different. She also remembers being told not to speak Urdu or Punjabi in the community by strangers: *'When my parents came to England, it was a different country, not as broad minded as it is now. I remember going into a shop or a chippy and speaking in Urdu to my parents, and being told to speak English … I remember even people who were just bystanders, who were just eavesdropping, would ask us to speak English. So English was forced on us, English was just "it"'.* Despite these experiences, as described earlier (see p.61), when she was around 11 Saadia decided to start speaking Urdu and wanting to be different seems to have played a large part in this decision. *'Speaking Punjabi wasn't anything special to me, it was normal, everybody spoke it. … But when I spoke Urdu, I used to love the fact that people couldn't tell that I was born here – I speak as if I could have been brought up in India'.*

Conclusion

Perhaps surprisingly, the two interviewees (Camilla & Sylvia) who did experience a deeper and longer lasting concern about fitting in were only different from their peers in terms of language and national origin, not in terms of ethnicity or religion. Both were girls. Both were in migrant families. Some of the other interviewees actually had much more negative experiences of racism or marginalisation (for example Vera W, as described above, or Mohammed above, and also p.146). Marion had also had some difficulty with this whilst at school in London, but this was resolved for her when her family moved to Cardiff in Wales when she was 10 years old (for more on this see p.111). Vera's experience also improved through a change of school. Each of these interviewees might have had longer lasting concerns if their context had not changed. None of these four women – Camilla, Sylvia, Marion or Vera W – has chosen to raise their child(ren) bilingually. I suspect that this may not be a coincidence.

- More interviewees had concerns whilst they were children about fitting in than did not, which suggests that most parents should expect this to come up at some point.
- However, in the vast majority of cases, these concerns were either minor or transitory or both. Some interviewees reacted by changing accents or to different extents downplaying or not advertising the fact that they spoke other languages. Parents may need to be sensitive to this. For example, to be prepared for a child to be embarrassed if a parent speaks to them in a minority language at school.
- From the tone of the interviewees' comments these concerns may well have been no more significant to the child concerned than other types of differences that children commonly experience at school (e.g. concerns about being tall/small, overweight/scrawny, having red hair/freckles, or being a teacher's pet or a 'nerd').
- Parents may face a choice between either downplaying the difference between their families and their children's peer group or else doing their utmost to raise their children with pride that they are different.

Of course, it is also possible to introduce your child to another peer group of children just like them – whether at a Saturday language school or just through meeting up with other multilingual families. They do not even need to speak the same language as you do (as we can attest from the reactions of the children attending our group in North London where the only thing that they have in common is that they are multilingual). Even if this peer group is secondary in that they do not spend as much time as they do with the children at school, it can still be hugely significant in reassuring children that they are not 'abnormal'.

Depending on where you live, it may well be case that far more children that your child meets and plays with are in fact multilingual than you are aware of. This is because many people who are multilingual are relatively shy about this and do not advertise the fact to all and sundry. In most countries, the school will have full details of all the languages that children speak at home, and without singling children out, there can be opportunities to celebrate children's home languages at school. In the UK there is an initiative called Multilingual Month, which is run each March (for a booklet of ideas for events on this see www.medway.gov.uk/docs/final_mmm_booklet_7.11.04.doc).

- Alternatively, many schools are running activities linked to a 'Language of the Month' throughout the year. There is an excellent website run by a primary school in Redbride in North East London which is a great resource for teachers and parents on this (see http://www.newburypark.redbridge.sch.uk/langofmonth/).
- It is possible to talk through with children why some children at school may tease or bully others. In some countries, children in schools will discuss this regularly. Children can understand from a surprisingly young age that other children bully because they themselves lack confidence and are unsure of themselves. Whilst this may not necessarily make it less hurtful if a child is picked on because they stand out for some reason, it can mean that the child is able to rise above it (which can disarm the bully who is not getting the reaction that they hoped for).
- Although we might associate the issue of 'not belonging' with migration, and some interviewees, such as Camilla, explicitly did so, even families whose ancestors had lived in their homes for generations but who spoke long-established minority languages such as Occitan reported feeling that they did not altogether fit in. It is interesting that Matilde felt that she fitted in fine whilst living in Africa (as a high-status immigrant) and felt more different from her peers in Italy with whom she shared nationality, ethnicity and a common language (possibly because she was returning from a continent with a low status in Italy).
- If you yourself feel self-conscious about 'not fitting in' where you are living, try not to communicate this to your children.
- Do not worry if your children want to downplay their multilingualism, they may have encountered jealousy from others, or just not want to draw attention to it in public. However, do keep reminding them how proud you are of them and their ability to speak more than one language in private.
- If your child is very sensitive to fitting in, a multilingual school may provide a very good answer for you. Some but not all of these are both fee-paying and expensive, and most but not all are located in capital or other cities, but if this is possible for you, it can make a big difference to sensitive children – see Claudia and Sylvia's comments above, p. 92–93.
- As your children get older (i.e. late teens or young adults) their peer group's reaction may switch to one of jealousy. Again you may be able to help prepare them for this – although it is difficult as you can either advise them to downplay their languages or else get them to see that someone being jealous is, in fact, hugely flattering.

13 Input from Others, Resources and Holidays

This chapter considers the influence of a number of factors wider than the nuclear family, which can be very important in a multilingual childhood. I cover the wider family, nannies and other child carers, holidays, books, films, TV and music, and organised religious activities.

Grandparents, Aunts, Uncles, Other Relatives, Godparents

When at WFBG we ask at our workshops with parents raising children multilingually *why* they want their children to be able to speak more than one language, one of the first and the most common responses is so that the children can communicate with grandparents and the wider family. In some migrant families, interviewees were no longer able to see their grandparents or other extended family, and for the children who learned a language through school, this is not relevant. However, for the remainder it is clear that grandparents and the wider family had significant impacts on many of our interviewees.

We have discussed above some examples where interviewees lived in extended families with their parents and grandparents (Sophie, p.25, Marion p.19, and Josune p.67) and clearly in these cases the grandparents had considerable influence in terms of the languages spoken by the children.

Even where they were not living together, grandparents often visited the interviewees and some stayed for quite lengthy periods. So Armelle's Argentinean grandparents would visit her in Europe for several months at a time. During these visits, although her grandparents did speak some French, Armelle would speak to them in Spanish (which was probably very helpful as at this time, as she preferred to reply to her Spanish-speaking mother in French, see p.86). Sometimes such visits would mean that the normal language pattern within the family was altered. So, in Markus's normally very flexible English and German-speaking household, when his German-speaking grandmother visited the family in the United States for several weeks the family changed their usual mixed-language pattern to German-only in order to communicate with the grandmother. *'That was very important to have a purely German period during that time [when living in the US when his German was weaker] to **have** to speak German'*. He also recalls her helping him with his reading and writing in German (as she was a primary schoolteacher).

In Helen's case (Dutch mother, English father), her mother would switch into speaking more English (the language Helen preferred not to speak, see p.83) during the visits of Helen's paternal English grandmother and other family who did not speak any Dutch. Helen's English grandmother would visit at least once a year and the family would visit England to see relatives. None of the English side of the family could speak any Dutch, and so the children always spoke English with their English extended family. Helen's mother would switch to mostly speaking English to the children when the English family were there – although she would still use Dutch if she found it easier. Helen remembers her grandmother commenting positively on the children's bilingualism: *'She would correct our [English] grammar sometimes but not in a negative way – she would suggest another way of saying something'.*

Ingrid recounted the efforts of her grandmother in the United States to support her English (growing up in Sweden) in some detail. As a very young child, until she was around two years old, Ingrid had lived in Mexico where she had learnt Spanish and had not spoken English or Swedish, although these were the languages that her parents had started out speaking to her. Ingrid thinks that her grandmother may have realised when she returned from Mexico speaking only Spanish that there was a risk that she would not speak English. *'When I came back from Mexico and could speak only Spanish I think my grandmother found that really frustrating'.* As a result, her grandparents seemed to value Ingrid's English and especially encouraged her to read in English. Ingrid would write letters and send postcards to her grandparents from Sweden. Ingrid remembers that her US grandparents were very supportive – during the holidays her grandmother would take her to the library to choose books in English and would also send her English tapes. Her grandfather would help her learn to spell words off by heart and test her on these.

One other interviewee who had been involved in a German Saturday school said of some of the children attending the school, *'A lot of them came from families where one partner was English one partner was German. It wasn't easy to keep up German language. It became an issue with grandparents… It was seen as really important'.* This suggests that, in these families, grandparents who spoke the children's minority language were very keen that their grandchildren maintained their bilingualism.

In other cases, the extended families of migrants had all moved to the UK. This provided opportunities for children to get together and speak the language with family members. Thus uncles, aunts, neighbours and tenants had a positive influence on raising Antony bilingually. In Vera W's case, her mother generally shied away from other Chinese people in England because of problems that she had had before she left China. Vera's family had some relatives in the UK and in America but they were unable to visit China, and for many years they had no or very sporadic contact with their family in China. There were, however, many occasions in the UK such as weddings where everyone who attended spoke Cantonese. She remembers adults spending hours playing mah-jong. There was an old friend of the family, who was a generation older than her parents, who was a little like a grandmother to Vera. When Vera's parents went away, Vera would go and stay with her. She spoke much less English than Vera's parents and Vera absolutely had to speak Cantonese to her.

However, even at family gatherings and weddings which were exclusively attended by people from one linguistic community, some interviewees told us that the languages used by children depended on which generation they were speaking to. For example, Saadia's family had a wide network of Punjabi-speaking family, friends and relatives in the area and they got together frequently. Family members would arrange religious ceremonies at people's houses. At these events the children were expected to speak Punjabi to adults; switching into English when speaking to adults at these events was not acceptable, although with relatives and friends their own age, the children would speak in English. In Mohammed's case, although he did not have a wide extended family in the UK, they were visited by members of the Bengali community and speaking good Bengali was very important. Mohammed remembers that it was very important that the children spoke Sylheti/Bengali (without an English accent) when the family did have Bengali visitors. Being able to speak Sylheti/Bengali well was an indication that children were being raised 'properly', not just in terms of their ability to speak a language but much more broadly. This was a source of pride and some status for the whole family, and visitors would comment on the children's good Bengali.

Occasionally, grandparents were slightly less supportive of parents' efforts to raise children bilingually. In Armelle's case, her mother spoke to her exclusively in Spanish, and her French mother-in-law, who did not speak Spanish, did not appreciate this. Armelle's mother would speak French to this side of the family although she continued to speak Spanish to her children, despite the remonstrations of her mother-in-law. *'When we went to our grandmother's country house and we were 15 cousins all together, my grandmother would say "Speak in French" but my mother always continued to speak Spanish to us – but I liked that. When my mother speaks to me in French ... her voice changes ... My grandmother is very French, closed, not very open, my mother was the only foreigner in the family'.*

Grandparents and other relatives of bilingual children in mixed-language households sometimes fear that if a child is raised speaking two languages and theirs is the child's weaker language, this will interfere with their relationship with the child. If they can (and sometimes even if they cannot...) they may try to talk to the child in his or her stronger language, in the hope that this will help them form a closer relationship. This is extremely frustrating for the parents of the child who may well have hoped to have a concentrated period of input in the child's weaker language during the holidays to help strengthen it. This whole issue is complicated by the fact that in many cases, the grandparents who speak the weaker language are physically removed from the children, and may see them less frequently. However, in our sample, many of the interviewees had established and maintained very strong relationships with grandparents and other relatives who were at a distance usually through visits. In fact (although interviewees did not usually explicitly make these comparisons, and sadly we had not had enough foresight to ask outright), reading into their tone of voice and choices of phrase, it seemed to us that, more often than not, interviewees seemed to be emotionally closer to those relatives who lived further away, who they had spent less time with and who spoke the minority language. Only one interviewee had any experience that supported these concerns that grandparents sometimes have. Camilla, who was a very shy child, mentioned that, *'I felt sometimes that I had a slightly stilted relationship with [my Danish grandparents] because I was slightly shy of speaking to them in Danish'.* In contrast, Armelle, in discussing her decision to live as an adult in Argentina, said: ' *... I chose Argentina because I am close to my extended family there. In Argentina I miss the culture in France but Argentina is very emotional and warm, whereas I feel that my French [extended] family is colder'.*

Although there is not the same emotional relationship, many families had visitors from a home country who brought both language and culture into the household. In some cases, this seems to have been a quite deliberate policy, whereas in other cases it may just have been the family being hospitable. One example of the former is Aimee who had moved aged eight from Togo to live in France with her aunt, who mainly spoke Kabye to her. The home was open to students who were coming from Togo to study in France, and Aimee's aunt welcomed these students through her networks in Togo and they not only came speaking Togolese languages (mainly Kabye) but also maintained the children's link with Togo.

One very important benefit of such visitors is that they bring up-to-date phrases and usage to the children. As languages change over time, many of our interviewees who were more isolated from the home country described their language sounding old-fashioned when they finally returned to these countries as adults. The more contact that children have with speakers who are immersed in the day-to-day development of language, and who are up to date in the latest phrases, slang and usages, the less likely this was to be the case (see also Chapter 27 where I discuss this issue along with that of whether or not the interviewees had accents).

Nannies and Other Child Carers

In our sample, we found only two examples where a nanny or childcare had had a particular influence on the interviewee's language. (We are excluding interviewees who learnt the basics of a language from childcare at a very young age – up to four and lost it again when input ceased – there were several examples of this.) Daniela had learnt French at her boarding school in Switzerland, and her mother arranged to have French au pairs after Daniela returned to England to an English school, which Daniela feels was good for her French.

A more detailed example is that of Parvati, who grew up in Britain speaking a mixture of Hindi and English with her mother and English with her father. Thus it was easy for her to add English words into Hindi sentences because both her parents spoke and understood English well. Even during regular trips to India, most people in her family could speak English, and only her grandmother could not. However, Parvati had nannies or au pairs throughout her childhood; some were English, some Swedish, and some Indian. She recalls that several times she had long-term Hindi-speaking nannies who did not speak much English. And she noticed the difference in that she needed to speak exclusively in Hindi if they were to understand, and she feels that this really helped to strengthen her Hindi. One in particular that Parvati remembers was with the family for several years when Parvati was already around 12 years old. *'This was really when I kind of forced myself to communicate with them [in Hindi] in ways that I had not needed to do with my family before'.* (Another reason that this was important to Parvati was that her mother moved 200 miles away for work reasons when Parvati was 10 or 11 and commuted between there and the family. She was no longer around every day and as Parvati's father spoke to his children in English, this nanny was Parvati's main source of Hindi.)

Holidays

Some interviewees had the opportunity to visit a country where their minority language was the majority language, which I will call an immersion holiday.

For some of our interviewees these trips seem to have been particularly important. In Ingrid's case (living in Sweden and hearing English from her mother, although Ingrid herself only spoke to her mother in Swedish – see p.83), each summer the family would go for long holidays to the United States to stay with relatives and see friends. Given that Ingrid spoke very little English herself in Sweden, these visits, and the English that Ingrid spoke during them, may have been important both in maintaining her active English as well as in helping reassure her mother that she could still, in fact, speak English when she needed to.

For Christine, her visits to her grandparents and wider family were crucial in her retaining her German because (as discussed on p.57) Christine's mother had been advised to stop speaking German to her children when Christine was around six years old. After this point in time, Christine's mother spoke only French to her; her father was French and the family lived in France. At that time there was no video and no chance of German TV or films, and so Christine's input in German whilst at home was extremely limited – in fact, more or less non-existent. The family went to stay with relatives in Germany at least once each year and sometimes twice, and they would occasionally stay several weeks. Christine did not have cousins, but had uncles who did not speak much French, as well as grandparents who did not speak any French, and she maintained her German almost entirely through these periodic visits.

Similarly, although for different reasons, Daniela's visits as a young child to her (divorced) father's family in Italy were equally important in her retaining Italian. She told us that she was only exposed to Italian whilst she was on these visits in Italy. She remembers when at the age of four she went back to Italy to stay with her father on her own for the first time after the divorce, and it was a traumatic experience (*'I want my mummy!'*). When she saw him she spoke to him in English. *'He was **very** keen to get me back into speaking Italian'.* Her grandparents and her cousins in Italy were always speaking Italian around her when she was there as a small child.

Like Ingrid, one interviewee had been so immersed in one language for two months that she initially struggled to speak her other language when she returned. Sabina recalls one particular visit when she was about eight when she and her mother went to visit Pakistan for around two months. *'Because I was immersed in the Urdu language, I do remember coming back and forgetting my English. It is something that has stuck in my mind. I remember my brother laughing at me …and telling me that I had forgotten my English'.*

For Sarah, even though she spoke German with her mother at home, she used to visit her mother's family in Germany during holidays and her German would quickly improve during this time. She used to buy German comics while on her visits, and she would stock up on these as they did not have them in Switzerland.

One interviewee (Antony) mentioned the fact that he was regarded as a wonder whilst on holiday in his small Cypriot village because as a small child he could count in both English and Greek.

Sylvia, who was living in France with English-speaking parents, also visited England regularly. These visits were mostly positive but she does remember some differences that were not just about language: at one party, for instance, she first encountered marmite in sandwiches (which she was expecting to be chocolate), which was swiftly followed by peanut butter (which she was expecting to be honey). And Sylvia was also the interviewee who, as quoted in the chapter above about fitting in and standing out, rather poignantly said, *'In the summer I was the French girl in England, and the rest of the year I was the English girl in France'.*

It certainly seems to be significant that all the interviewees who talked about these immersion holidays as particularly positive or significant would generally have travelled at least once a year and normally described the holidays as 'long', clearly in many cases at least several weeks, sometimes several months. Interviewees who travelled in this way only every two or three years or even less frequently than that seemed to feel that the visits had had much less impact.

Books, Films, TV, Music

Some of our interviewees had access to books in their minority language, but not all. Some did not learn to read in that language. Many remembered being read to in various languages by their parents (but, again, not all). In her family with a strict 'English only at home rule', Sylvia remembers that every day during the long school lunch break they would read to/with their mother in English, and later, when they could read well, would read English books on their own until it was time to go back to school. Ingrid in Sweden remembers learning to read in Swedish, although her mother read to her a lot in English at home. Camilla remembers having Danish books, which she loved. In Adeyinka's case (he grew up in Nigeria speaking Yoruba at home and English at school), all of his friends were also reading a lot in English and they would talk about the books that they had read. In contrast, the only books available in Yoruba were the textbooks that they studied at school and Adeyinka has never read in Yoruba beyond these. Other interviewees read books in a language only whilst on holiday in a country where that was the majority language, so Helen, the child of an English father and a Dutch mother living in Holland, would start to read a book in English during a holiday in England but would not continue to read and to finish the book when she returned to Holland.

Films were less important to our interviewees than one suspects they would be to bilingual children growing up today, and many interviewees did not mention them or, when asked, said that they were not available. One notable exception to this was the Bollywood films watched by all of the children who spoke Hindi and Urdu. So, Parvati and her mother and sister would quite often watch a Bollywood movie in the afternoon whilst Parvati's mother embroidered the border on a sari, and Parvati feels that she learnt a lot of Hindi from those movies. Vera W remembers watching soap operas in Cantonese when staying with a cousin (who was her parents' age). In contrast, her parents did not get any Chinese videos and the family watched English TV. Of course, in mixed-language families where one parent does not understand the language the other uses to speak to the children, watching films or listening to music in that language may be more problematic. In Sarah's family, her father did not speak or understand German, and Sarah thinks her mother would have liked to have watched more German films with them, but the family's common language was English. Sarah feels as a result that she does not know much about 'German cultural icons' or books which German children read.

Parvati was one of the few interviewees who mentioned parents singing to them as children, as her mother used to *'sing to us [in Hindi] to put us to sleep and I still know all of those songs....'*.

In Fatima's case, the TV was an important resource for her to start to learn the new majority language when she arrived in the UK aged 10 from Morocco. Her parents worked in a hotel, and for the first year the children did not go to school but stayed in the hotel and watched a lot of TV, which was important in helping them to pick up some English. *'We watched TV. I remember watching Playschool and we would sit and listen and pick up language. The first word I picked up was the word "people". I was fascinated by this word "people", it sounded so strange to me ... I used to go round saying "Hello people, hello people" ... call my Dad "People Dad". We were fascinated by the accent, it sounded **so** strange. We were used to French with its sounds "en", that kind of sound and English sounded so different. I know people say that TV is bad, but we learnt quite a lot from watching TV, listening ... absorbing'.*

Religious Activities

In many cases there was not a particular religion associated with a language. Some interviewees' parents were not religious at all. In some cases both linguistic communities (whether mixed-language families or immigrant families in host communities) followed the same religion. Just as our sample contained no examples of mixed-race families, there were also no examples of mixed-religion families. This is almost certainly again a function of the fact that all of the interviewees were at least 18 years old and relationships across religions were much less common a few decades ago.

However, there were examples where religion was associated with one language and was an important factor either in the parents' motivation for children being bilingual, or in children being exposed to one or other language.

Parvati's mother was very concerned that the children should develop a very good knowledge of Hindi culture and religious traditions. They followed the religious traditions at home; however, the family did not attend a Hindu temple and so were not part of a Hindi-speaking community through their religion. *'My mum taught us to pray in Hindi when we were very little girls. I still pray today [in Hindi]… when I need to relax, for example, if I am on a plane and I need to sleep. It reminds me of being young and going to bed'.*

Like Parvati, Saadia's family were also religious, but they also organised religious activities within the family and Saadia did not go to a Mosque until she was an adult. The case of Muslim interviewees is a little more complex because the language of Islam is always Arabic, and some of those we interviewed with an Islamic background spoke Urdu or Bengali. This was not the case for Saad, who was bilingual in Arabic and Kurdish. Saad grew up when there was considerable tension between the Kurdish and Arab community in Iraq. The fact that his father was a devout Muslim, a professor of Islamic studies, and was proud to speak excellent Arabic as the language of Islam, may have helped Saad to have a positive attitude to both his languages in this polarised situation. As his father had started teaching Saad the Koran as a small child, this meant that he did speak and understand some Arabic when he started primary school, although, until then, apart from this religious input, his family had spoken to him exclusively in Kurdish.

Several interviewees speaking Asian languages learnt to recite Koranic verses in Arabic, but Mohammed learnt Arabic as a fourth language in a much more complete way. His parents arranged a private Arabic tutor for their children who taught them for two and a half hours each week. The children were taught to talk and understand Arabic as well as to read, recite and understand the Koran. Mohammed remembers his father sacking one of these teachers because he felt he was ignorant. Arabic was important for religious reasons. *'Learning Arabic, I felt, was actually more important than learning Bengali, because to be a Muslim ignorant of the holy book's language was profoundly disturbing'.*

For Susanne, religion was intimately bound up with language because her father was the pastor of a German-language church. The family spoke German at home and in the church community, which also included a German Saturday school for children (see p.131 for more on this school).

Marion, who grew up with English and Welsh in a polarised family situation and who initially struggled at school, commented that there was also a Methodist Welsh church in London which she thinks could have been used as a place where she could have received some support. Unfortunately her parents did not go to this church because it was too far away. Marion sees church as a good place of support for bilingual children, especially if their languages have been marginalised.

Conclusion

It is clear that all these wider sources of support were very important to different interviewees growing up bilingually. No interviewee benefitted from all of them and different factors were important to different people.

- In our sample, wider families, particularly grandparents, stood out as significant. Grandparents (especially if they are monolingual) are important in providing motivation to both parents and children to maintain a language that enables a relationship between children and their grandparents. Grandparents also often provided significant childcare whether regularly or during longer holidays, which was an opportunity for language input. Most grandparents on both sides were very supportive.
- Our sample did not suggest that interviewees were emotionally closer to or had better relationships with grandparents who lived closer to them or who were speakers of a child's stronger language or the majority language where they lived. Only one interviewee felt that there had been a language barrier between her and one set of her grandparents.
- If your parents or parents-in-law are concerned about this, show them this section of this book or summarise it for them, and explain to them that the best way to form a really strong relationship with the child is to communicate with them, and that they will communicate best when they speak their most fluent language to their grandchildren.
- Other visitors to your household can be a very useful influence. If they are travelling from abroad to visit you, they may help your children to keep up to date with the latest slang, phrases, idioms and vocabulary for new products/software and so on in a setting where the language is the majority language. Otherwise there is a risk that your children will speak a perfectly fluent and accentless language, which sounds incredibly old-fashioned or dated.
- Nannies, au pairs or childminders can be a very useful form of support for a language within the household. This may be particularly the case if the nanny is a monolingual speaker of a child's weaker language or the language that they do not use at school. It was also very important in some families where other forms of input had ceased, or were reduced or temporarily interrupted for reasons of career or divorce.
- Another very important factor for our interviewees was regular immersion holidays to a country where a child's minority language is a majority language. These trips are worth their weight in gold. Go for as long as you can. Try to go at least once a year if you can. In our sample, those who travelled only once every three or four years reported a much lower impact. Arrange for your children to spend time with monolingual children if you can (or, if this is not possible, any monolingual speakers).
- The links between language and religion were much less common or developed than I would have expected. They were important for some interviewees, but even then, were often organised within the immediate or extended family rather than through an external community at a mosque, church or temple. Some other research seems to suggest that having a specific place or community where one language is spoken exclusively can also be important in sustaining bilingualism and organised religious activities, and communities certainly provide this. So it was perhaps surprising that we did not find more examples of religion linked with language learning.

- From our conversations at the WFBG, it seems to me that today's generation of parents may set much store on the availability of books, songs, films and TV in several languages. However, few of our interviewees remembered these as particularly significant factors, although, when prompted, some mentioned reading in various languages. Two interviewees remembered enjoying reading comics. Two interviewees remembered Bollywood films. Several interviewees recalled viewing films, music, or books in English in their teenage years as being 'cool', which had an influence on their willingness to speak English.
- Essentially, if as a parent you need to choose between buying a bilingual library of books, CDs and DVDs or in paying for a ticket for a holiday (preferably with monolingual family members) in another country where a minority language is the majority or only language, I would go for the holiday. I would also try to make such holidays as regular as possible; try to make sure that they are very enjoyable for the children and, once the children are old enough, I would try to find ways to leave the child(ren) with trusted relatives or friends there in a monolingual environment, if possible for at least a week, and preferably longer.
- Some children may temporarily find it difficult to speak their other language(s) on their return home if they have just been immersed in a monolingual language environment for a while. Do not worry, this will soon pass. Just do not arrange for them to do a drama audition for a desperately longed for part in a play in the language that they may struggle in on their first day back…
- I am not sure what you can do about cultural misunderstandings like mistaking marmite for chocolate. If you visit the destination country frequently you may be able to taste most traditional foods whilst you are there, or bring traditional foods from your country back with you so that your child is initiated into the culture of cuisine (and into as many other facets of cultural life as possible).

PART 3

Education

14 Starting School and Changing Schools

15 Home Language Support/Teaching in
Mainstream Schools

16 Additional Support Outside (or as an
alternative to) Mainstream Schools

17 Help with Homework

A concern which frequently arises in families who speak one language at home and another in the community is that their children will not speak enough of the majority language to get on well at school. This section explores our interviewees' recollections of their school days. Many were in the situation of starting at a school using as a medium a language that the child did not speak at home. We have divided these into those who did this when they were less than seven years old, and those who moved schools later in their childhoods as the issues (and conclusions) are different. We then discuss the support available at school for a few lucky children in some countries for home languages (primarily in Sweden). Far more children attended beginners' foreign language classes in a language that they already spoke at home. Their experiences in these classes were very mixed indeed and are set out next. I move on to discuss home education very briefly as we had no interviewee in our sample who was educated at home instead of attending school. However, many interviewees who grew up in the UK had attended Saturday language schools and this leads into a discussion about interviewees learning to read and write in two or more languages. And finally in this part of the book, I look at what interviewees' parents did about helping children with their homework – as this a very common issue of concern for parents of multilingual children at the age when they start to bring home significant amounts of work from school.

14 Starting School and Changing Schools

Many, many parents (as well as teachers and education policy-makers) worry that if children start school in a language that they do not fully understand and speak fluently (for their age), the children will miss out, fall behind and never catch up. This is, in our experience, one of the most common reasons that parents in multilingual families give for deciding not to raise children bilingually. Parents who do want their children to be bilingual also sometimes start speaking the majority language to them when they are around four or five years old to try to ease their transition into the majority language at school – which can often be the start of a process whereby the majority language is used more and more, and the minority language less and less at home.

Just over half of our interviewees either started in or moved into a school that used a language they did not speak at home. The vast majority of our interviewees suffered absolutely no short-term, let alone long-term, disadvantage from doing so. Of the 18 interviewees who started at nursery or at the beginning of primary school (i.e. aged around five or six) using a language not spoken at home, 15 reported no problems at all, and all but one adjusted to school in a new language within weeks or months. So only three interviewees remembered having had *any problems at all* and only one interviewee remembered those problems continuing longer than a couple of months. In fact, for those interviewees living in a community that spoke that language (but who spoke another language at home), it seems that the passive knowledge that they had picked up very informally from interactions in the community as very young children was quite high. But all this applies to those starting school in nursery, reception or at least the very first few years of school; the later that interviewees started school where the medium was a language they did not speak or understand, the more likely they were to report either short-term or longer-term difficulties. Two interviewees could be considered to have been in some way disadvantaged in the long term by their relatively late switch in the language of schooling; one moved school when she was seven (but her schooling was also later very disrupted by her mother's health problems), and the other child moved when she was 10 and missed one year of school entirely. One interviewee who moved aged 11 to Australia put in a great deal of effort and eventually succeeded, although he found this quite tough. Another interviewee who moved when she was 12 to Sweden did not feel that her education was adversely affected in any way.

Starting School in a New Language – When the Interviewees were Under Seven Years Old

Fifteen out of eighteen interviewees who had this experience said that, for a variety of reasons, this presented them with no problems. All of these interviewees started their schools very early. Some went into a nursery or preschool system at around three or four and the rest went into a first primary school class between the ages of four and six.

Some, although speaking one minority language at home, had had enough input from the community and preschool clubs and playgroups to have a working knowledge of the majority language. So, for example, Saadia's family lived in an area of England with many Punjabi speakers and Saadia would mix with the children of friends and neighbours who all spoke Punjabi, but those children who were going to school also spoke English and, in fact, amongst themselves seemed to prefer to speak English. Before she started school, Saadia had a passive knowledge of English but could not speak it well. *'I remember when I was very young, everyone [i.e. the local children] would be in the garden and I would be sitting on this coal box and everyone would be chatting in English, but I was the only one who would have to talk in Punjabi, until my English was strong enough'.* Saadia remembers starting at nursery and then school with no problems, so by then she had acquired enough English to participate, although she also remembers that she was a very shy child and probably did not actively contribute very much in any language. Similarly, Susanne reported learning English in a playgroup by interacting with other children, and we mentioned earlier how Saad's Kurdish father had started teaching him Arabic through the Koran before he went to an Arabic-medium school. In four cases, the interviewees went into bilingual schools, which, in most cases, made special provision to help children become proficient in the language they did not speak at home (see Chapter 3 Interviewees who are Bilingual Solely through Attending School in Another Language p.38). Even Snjezana in an Italian language-medium school in Croatia, where no special arrangements were made for the children who did not speak Italian at home (like her), found that she quickly gained a good command of the language (and indeed soon went on to rival the mother-tongue Italian speakers).

In Sweden as a preschool child, Ingrid spoke more English than Swedish, and her mother arranged for her to complete two years of her first year of school by starting one year early to ensure that her Swedish was good enough to understand the lessons so that she would not be disadvantaged in any way. Other interviewees simply reported that they experienced no problems when they started school or nursery. So, again we have already covered (p.92) Camilla's switch from speaking only Danish to only English when she started at nursery. Within a very short time, Camilla was very fluent in English – with just the occasional mistake with an idiomatic phrase, which I suspect many other people would not have been aware of.

In Bindi's case, she recalls speaking mostly Gujarati with English words occasionally interspersed in Gujarati sentences at home. At around three years old, Bindi attended an English-medium nursery where she started hearing English systematically and learnt to speak it. The nursery staff did not speak Gujarati although many of the other children were Asian and would have done so. Bindi does not recall any problems being understood in English at nursery and believes that her parents had taught her enough English before she went to nursery school so that she could understand and make herself understood.

In our sample, compared to the 15 who reported absolutely no problem at all, there were three interviewees who found the linguistic aspects of school or nursery initially more difficult even though they too started school early. For two interviewees these problems were very quickly resolved and they had no long-term impact. Only one interviewee had more lasting problems that were only resolved after a change of both place and school when the interviewee was around nine years old.

Sylvia was one of the two interviewees who remembered problems that were resolved quickly. She grew up in an English family in France, and started preschool aged around three. At this point Sylvia could speak very little French and she does have clear memories of trying to make herself understood at school and not being able to get across what she wanted to say. She recalls, for example, being asked by the teacher what she had had for lunch (at home) and she did not know the word in French, so she guessed or made it up and the teacher did not understand her. She also recalls the class being given instructions in French that she did not understand. Despite recalling incidents like these, her recollection of her early school life is positive and she does not remember any problems with teachers or other children as a result of her limited French in the early months at school.

Similarly, Vera W's parents spoke exclusively in Cantonese to their children; Vera also had a Cantonese-speaking nanny when she was very small, and as a very small child, Vera was a monolingual Cantonese speaker. Vera was the last of four children and her siblings were 11, 9 and 6 years older than her. When Vera was a toddler, her sisters spoke English to her to try to teach her the language. Vera thinks that this was so that when she started kindergarten she would understand more. *'I remember them sitting me down and pointing to things and telling me the words in English'.* Despite this, when Vera started attending a private nursery school, she found that she could not understand what was happening – she found the whole experience very alien and, as a result, she did not like going and did not like her mother leaving her there.

Marion

One case really stands out as being unusual and of concern, and that is the case of Marion, a Welsh/English bilingual child who started school in London. Marion actually spoke English at home with her mother and grandfather, as well as Welsh with her father and grandmother, and so was not strictly speaking a child who started school in a language she did not understand. She does say that at this stage she was probably more comfortable speaking Welsh, as her mother was working and her father and grandmother spent more time with her. Marion's problem seems to have been that when she spoke she used quite a lot of Welsh, and may well have mixed Welsh with English in the same sentences. She seems to have had a particular issue with reading and writing and this is clearly bound up with language. Marion said: *'It was difficult in school, I did not get on and I was not considered very bright at all in school, and I had a particular difficulty with reading. My father insisted that I learnt to read in Welsh. He was teaching me to read in Welsh. At the same time I was learning to read English in school. I was not able to read until I was 10, which is interesting because now I'm a professor of English literature [laughs]'*. In London her first teacher was very *'kind and understanding'*, and her first year at school was very *'gentle'*. Marion did all her sums in Welsh, and her maths was fine, although she was having difficulty in reading and writing. Her second teacher was much stricter. *'She was very sharp. I was not allowed to speak any Welsh at all. I think I was the only [Welsh-speaking child] in the whole school. I was given the example of my sister who hadn't had any problems at all. I always felt that I was the one who was not as clever as my sister'*. (Marion's sister had primarily been raised by her mother who preferred to speak English, and so her sister did not speak very much Welsh at all. For more on this unusual family, see p.19.)

Marion's grandparents died while she was in London and her father got a new job in Cardiff. She celebrated her tenth birthday in Wales. *'Moving back to Wales was a major breakthrough for me'*. Her new teacher was a Welsh/English bilingual and Marion quickly learned to read. *'From September when I started school to the end of the following summer I became top of my class. I'd gone in as a special needs child and [came out] with the highest mark. ... I realise now that I must have been learning all that time, but refused to show any of it. I must have been learning to read, because the first book I read in English was Charles Kingsley's Westward Ho, which is an immensely heavy text for a child to read. Now there was a teacher who could speak to me in my own kind of pidgin language. She turned me around! Also being in an environment where I wasn't mocked, where I was considered "normal".... There was sufficient bilingualism around to give you a feeling that it was OK. Many teachers were bilingual'*.

Marion adds: *'I always tell people with children who are either bilingual or multilingual that if they do have difficulty with reading, not to worry because they will come to it. I give myself as an example of success because I "could not read", I was a "backward" child, I was in the special learning group in school until I got to 10 when I suddenly was reading. ...In my experience, the negative attitude of teachers to bilingualism really puts you back'*.

Starting School in a New Language – When the Interviewees were Seven Years Old or Over

The four cases where interviewees switched the language they spoke at school when they were slightly older were all remembered in detail by the interviewees, and half of these interviewees reported more problems than the interviewees who started or switched at younger ages.

Mumtaz

Mumtaz left Pakistan when she was seven years old. In Pakistan she had completed a year of basic education in Urdu. When she started at the local English primary school:

'It was very difficult … floods of tears, I didn't understand what people were saying around me so I thought that they were talking about me and I was thinking "What are they planning?" I didn't understand a word. … It was scary. … I came home every day in tears'. She thinks that she was very distressed for around a week before she began to settle down at school. Mumtaz had one-to-one language support for about half an hour twice a day for 20 or 30 minutes, which she found extremely helpful. Mumtaz remembers that she was given particular words to take home each day in a little metal tobacco box, *'our precious little boxes'.* She would read them with her father: *'He would help me and he would praise me. Once I had read them … he was pleased that I was learning English … he was pleased that I was picking it up, he would praise me every day'.* This language support continued throughout her primary education until she was around 10 or 11 and was much appreciated by Mumtaz: *'That was excellent, that was'.* In her early years at primary school, Mumtaz feels that she missed out on a lot of education because she could not understand enough English: *'At primary school, I missed out on a lot of things … science … because we didn't have the language so we missed out on everything that was happening. All those things that they were throwing at me …I didn't take in, because I didn't understand English'.* With very little input in English at home, Mumtaz recalls that it took about three years before her English was on a par with all the other children in her class and she could understand all of her lessons. By this time, she was in the last year of primary school.

Later in the interview Mumtaz mentioned that she felt that, in many ways, her younger brothers and sister, who were born in the UK, had life easier than her because she and her sister would speak English to them at home, so that they had some knowledge of English before they started school. (However, she also mentioned that these younger siblings are not confident speaking Urdu and much prefer speaking English today.) Mumtaz's experience is complicated by the fact that as a result of a family tragedy her mother was seriously depressed for much of Mumtaz's early childhood to the extent that she was not fully able to look after her children. Some of the burden of this fell on Mumtaz, so that she missed school when either her mother or one of her sisters or brothers was unwell. Clearly this had a significant impact on Mumtaz's progress at school and it is hard to separate out the impact that missing school had on her from the impact of her transition into the UK education system from Pakistan aged seven.

Fatima

Although Fatima found education in England a very positive experience, her education was probably the most disrupted by her parents move from Morocco to England when she was 10 years old. After the move, for about a year, Fatima and her brothers and sisters did not go to school at all. When she did start school, in East London in the mornings she went with another group of children for two hours of language tuition for children who had limited English. This was a very small class and the teacher was able to do one-to-one work as well as group work. Fatima felt that this language support helped her a lot. She also had very supportive friends who would help her when she did not understand in the mainstream classes. School was positive, but she also says: *'The exams came fairly quickly and I didn't do too well in the exams – except French'.* Perhaps it is significant that none of Fatima's family spoke English – even her father who had spent some years in England before his family came to join him had not learnt the language. Also neither of Fatima's parents had themselves benefitted from an education as children in Morocco. Fatima also mentions that her younger sister who was five when she arrived in the UK *'did better academically than I did because she came into the system younger ...'.*

Tom

Tom moved from Croatia to Australia when he was 11 years old. His father was a skilled labourer. His parents could not speak any English, and prior to the move Tom only knew some basic words. He travelled with his family to Australia by ship, which he says felt like a holiday cruise. There were English lessons on the ship, but Tom did not bother going as there were interesting distractions on board, like a swimming pool and games with other children. Once they had arrived in Melbourne, Tom was enrolled in a local Catholic primary school. In Croatia, he had attended a state school, which gave him a good rounded education. He had completed year four and was one of the better students. Upon arrival in Australia he was put straight into year six because of his age, totally missing year five. The school did not provide any specific language support. It was pure immersion. He felt that he was just thrown in at the deep end. *'There was a boy in my class whose parents were originally from Croatia, but he was born in Australia. English was his first language, Croatian was his second language. I remember our class teacher, a nun, introducing me to the boy to make me a bit at ease, to have someone to talk to in my language'.* Tom did not understand the boy's Croatian very well at first, but they soon became very good friends. Tom started to pick up conversational English very quickly. Because language was not his strength, he shied away from language-based subjects. Spelling exercises were something new to him. *'I was very good at maths and science. That's how I dealt with it in the short term. I concentrated on what I felt comfortable with. I just bluffed my way through it and managed to get through year six quite well'.*

When he received a certificate at the end of year six, it gave him a real feeling of satisfaction that he had achieved something. It was challenging, but Tom did not mind this because his parents were very supportive. Although his parents did not have academic qualifications, they brought Tom up to believe that it was important to do well academically. The secondary school Tom went to had the same make up as the primary school. It was run by French-Canadian Christians. *'They all spoke English and French so they understood the problems of kids not being able to communicate'.* Tom now says: *'Language expression was always my weakest subject and I think I should have spent more time on it. I was doing enough to get through. You were left to your own resources to fend for yourself. There was nothing in the educational system to support these groups'.* He did his best and ended up as the fifth best performer for year seven. This made him realise that he was doing something right, although he was frustrated at times.

Particularly stressful was year 12, and the final exams: *'The three hours was spent primarily writing essays. I had heard many stories of kids failing and repeating the last year because they didn't pass English, and I just didn't want to be like that. Fortunately I did enough to get through. I worked very hard to achieve that. Reading was not my strength at that stage, I didn't read a lot of novels. I couldn't enjoy books. I remember buying little booklets summarising major literary works and reading them to make sure I understood fully the themes of the books. In the end it worked sufficiently to get through the exams'.* His secondary schoolteachers were mostly from non-English backgrounds. Tom remembers them as being tolerant and patient in class. *'It was probably the patience of the teachers that nurtured something there, at least allowed me to develop, to get me through'.* Tom now thinks it would have helped if he had had structured lessons in English away from the mainstream, and which fed into the mainstream in terms of English expression and literature.

Shadi

Shadi is the exceptional case in this small group of interviewees who moved at a later age. Despite the fact that she arrived in Sweden when she was 12, she very quickly learnt Swedish at her state school. This was her fourth move of country and language, as she had by this time also lived in Iran, England and France. *'When I started school in Sweden – I was 12 – all my friends spoke to me in English, ... and I didn't learn a word of Swedish for three months. But then I remember the head teacher had a big assembly one day, the whole school was there, and she said (first in English so that I could understand) "From this day on, nobody speaks in English to Shadi". And I also had a special teacher to teach me Swedish. And my friends stuck to this – they did speak Swedish. And after three months I could understand anything, after six months I was speaking fluently'.*

Moving to a School Using a Language You Already Know but Which You Have Not Used at School Before

In the above we have been discussing interviewees who attended schools that used a language that they did not speak or hear at home. It would be easy to assume that, in contrast, children would be able to move relatively easily between different schools using the various languages that they already speak. Seven interviewees in our sample moved between schools in this way. Certainly, being able to speak the language does avoid some of the issues described above, but several interviewees mentioned that their teachers or parents felt that they needed language support, or recalled that their written language skills were not at the standard needed for school. There were also more subtle differences of language use, syllabus and culture that they needed to cope with. Even interviewees who continued to use the same language as the medium of education but moved countries had some problems, which tells us that some of the issues attributed to changes of language may actually be due to other factors, different curriculums, different styles of teaching, different expectations and different standards.

Learning to Read and Write in French for the First Time Aged 11

Matilde is quite a straightforward example of a child who had learnt to talk and understand a language but who had never read or written in that language. She had already lived in what was then Zaire for two years when she was six. During this period, she did not attend any school as the family was in a very remote area where there was no school, but she was taught at home in Italian by her mother. She learnt French from playing with other children in the community and from the nanny/home help (see p.45). The family then returned to Italy for three years, where Matilde had almost no input in French apart from an occasional conversation with her brother or on rare occasions when the family met up with French speaking friends. After three years back in Italy, when Matilde was 11, the family returned to Zaire to live in a larger town. Matilde and her brother were to be admitted to a private Belgian school in the town which taught in French. *'I could talk and understand French. But I did have a problem with the writing – as I had never been taught to read or write in French'.* When they returned to Zaire, there was a month before school started and Matilde and her brother were sent to stay for two weeks with some French-speaking nuns. Matilde's mother also arranged for a local girl to come and talk to the children, and she went over the numbers and other words in French with them. But this girl was not a fully-qualified teacher, and Matilde felt that this was quite basic. In fact, despite the three-year gap in input, Matilde remembers that she had no problem understanding or talking in French as soon as they got back to Zaire. At the Belgian school, Matilde could understand everything and respond verbally in class, but she really struggled with the writing. *'I remember coming home on one of the first days and asking my Mum "What's that strange letter that they do which is an 'S' and a 'C' together?" It was an "X" but I didn't know what it was. I suffered a lot to learn to write French properly. … I remember the first dictation. The maximum mark was 20 and they would take a mark off for each mistake, and I got something like minus 20. I remember crying all day, that day. But I had a very good teacher, with good technique and he got me copying out words 40 times and by the end of the year, I got good marks in dictation'.*

Family Organising Additional Support

Claudia could already read and write in German when she moved aged around eight to a German-medium school, but her family felt that she needed support to get her German to a level where she could do well in a German-medium school. She says: *'I think my father at some points got worried because he thought my German was slipping …. So when I started going to German schools in England and Cairo, he spoke German to me a lot because I was in a German education system and had to get my German to a **perfect** level'.* She remembers it being a little difficult when she first started attending a German school in Germany. Her parents organised a tutor who gave her classes after school to help her get her German to a higher level. Despite this, she does not recall any other pupils commenting on any mistakes she made in German (although she does recall pupils making disparaging remarks about other things, including, for example, about the fact that she had been living in Africa). This suggests that, if anything, she probably needed help most with her reading and writing in German. She also does not recall teachers commenting on any problems, which suggests that her level of German, including her written German, was probably quite high and that her father was being particularly careful or had very high standards.

A Really Good Teacher

Of course, changing schools is about a lot more than language. Isabelle, whose parents divorced and whose experiences we discussed above (see p.51), actually switched school systems twice. The first time she was very unwilling to change country, language and school, but after some initial fears, she did not find language to be a problem. She had attended a bilingual French/English school in the United States until she was nine, but then moved into a French-medium school when she moved to France. This was at the time of her parents' divorce and she did not want to move at all. However, Isabelle was fortunate with her new teacher at her new French school. This teacher noticed that she was shy and made a point of introducing her to the other children in her class, and asked them all to make a special effort to welcome her as she had just come from America to live in France. *'My whole attitude was wrong. I didn't want to be there. I was very angry. But I was really lucky ... The French teacher was just lovely ... she made this formal introduction ... and at recess all of the kids were asking me these questions about America and I was the sensation. It was so bizarre because I had never experienced that in my life. It was lovely in a way, and I felt "it's OK, it's alright". I did very well at school that year'.* Clearly Isabelle's level of French from both her family and her bilingual school in the United States enabled her to understand and read and write well enough to do well in the French school system.

A Transition Year in a Bilingual School

Later on, Isabelle moved in the opposite direction from a French-medium school to an English-medium school. Despite a transition year in a bilingual English/French school in Belgium, the linguistic elements of this move were less straightforward – possibly because Isabelle was much older and the complexity and range of language used at this stage of education is much higher. By this point she was almost 16, and had spent over five years in the monolingual French school system with quite limited input in English. Her father took up an opportunity to take a year of work in Belgium and both Isabelle and her brother moved to live with him there. They were both enrolled in an international school that had a bilingual English and French stream. Isabelle had been speaking and hearing predominantly French for six years, and when she sat the tests to determine her level of English she did not do well and so was put in a class of French children who were learning English as a foreign language. She dealt with this during the first lesson by answering every single question that the teacher asked; at the end of the lesson she went to speak with the teacher who acknowledged that she was in the wrong group and she was moved. Isabelle feels that this transitional year in Belgium was very important to her being able to cope at the high school level, when she and her brother moved back to Atlanta to live with her father on a more permanent basis. She explains that she found it difficult and frustrating to write in English at this point. *'I went from the French education system to the American education system. I was actually very good at expressing myself in French. Literature was my forte. So suddenly having to express myself in English was really frustrating because all I could ever achieve was an approximation of what I wanted to say, whereas I knew that there was a perfect word… but it just didn't come to me in English'.* The situation was even more difficult for her brother who was five years younger than her and had left the United States for France before he could read or write, and this year in Belgium was when he learnt to read and write in English for the first time (aged around 13). Isabelle remembers her father sitting for long periods with her brother, working with him to help him get his English to a level where he would be able to cope in school in the United States. (This was successful and her brother went on to graduate with a university degree in the United States.)

Other interviewees, though, made similar transitions at similar ages with fewer problems or issues. Josune attended a Basque-medium school throughout her schooling until she reached university level. In terms of spoken language, Josune thinks she was a balanced bilingual by the age of ten. She also read Spanish and Basque fiction books. She did not write much in Spanish as all her schoolwork was in Basque. When she went to a Spanish university the transition was fairly smooth as she was already bilingual. She had to work on her writing, and for the first time she had to take notes in Spanish. Perhaps surprisingly, she found maths in Spanish quite a challenge as she was used to mathematical terminology in Basque. *'That was the most difficult area to understand'.*

Cultural as well as Linguistic Differences Between Schools in the Same City

Christopher's transition between schools using different languages was the least successful, although, in his case, he moved between schools in the same city. Although he had always lived in England and had mainly lived with his English father after the age of 10 when his parents separated, Christopher remembers struggling when he moved aged 15 from the French *lycée,* where he was taught in French and studied English only as a foreign language, to an English-medium secondary school. *'I never took to the English school. It was just too much to take in at that age. I didn't do the exams, I wasn't proficient, I couldn't get into the system'.* His younger brother, who had also gone to the French school and made the same switch at a younger age, managed to get through the exams. *'Because he was younger he was able to get into the system and pass the exams, and he went to university'.* There were other differences between the schools than language: *'I felt very much a foreigner. The lycée is mixed, boys and girls in the same classroom. The English school was boys only and that was a real shock, because whereas at fifteen you have a boyfriend or a girlfriend in the French school, here they were only starting to talk about girls, and didn't go beyond that. The boys were still giggling away… [laughs]'.*

Aimee also recalls problems switching school systems even though, in her case, she switched from a French-medium school in Togo to another French-medium school in France when she was eight. This was partly due to differences in the French used but also partly due to differences in the curriculum in the two settings: *'I remember when I came to France, the first class I was in, it was hard because the way that they spoke French in Togo and in France was different. … Sometimes they gave me some tests, … and I did not do well … it took me three months of working very hard at home to get from being the last in the class to being the best in the class. The vocabulary was different, the books were different … history and geography was different, we had learnt African history and geography … whereas maths was straightforward. … At home I had a lot of support to catch up. I did a lot of French grammar exercises at home … Every night several times a week, my uncle would mark the exercises that I had done and help me. My aunt paid for additional tuition from students for her children – and they allowed me to join these lessons'.* Despite the fact that she was transitioning between education systems only and not languages, Aimee feels that she benefitted greatly from this additional support.

Conclusion

Our interviews confirm that parents should not worry about children starting school in a language they do not speak at all or have a limited knowledge of at the start of primary school or earlier. Problems are particularly unlikely if the children have already lived in a place where the language used at a school is also used in the community.

The level of language that children starting primary school need to function in the first year classroom, follow what is going on, to learn and participate is quite limited. Children will learn this level of language very quickly if they are completely new to the language (as did Camilla). In fact, if they have already heard the language spoken at all, they may already be able to understand this level of the language from very limited initial input (as did Bindi and Saadia). If children do have some initial problems understanding and making themselves understood (e.g. Sylvia and Vera W), these will almost always pass very quickly. Marion was the only child who reported any medium-term problems and her case is actually different as it concerns a child who could already understand English when she started school in English. We have to hope that most teachers today would not deal with a bilingual child who seemed to be bright (i.e. she had no problem with her maths) but who was struggling to learn to read and write as Marion's second teacher did. The whole situation was compounded by explicit prejudice against the Welsh, which the school did not challenge (see p.147). It is hard not to wonder how Marion's story would have turned out had the family not moved to Wales when she was 10 years old. Marion herself told us, *'I think when they realised I was sinking at school, they should have either moved me to a school that had a Welsh component in it, or they should have hired a tutor. My father was very active at the London Welsh group and they could have used that to find somebody who would actually help me, or a support group. Maybe when I was little there wasn't a support group ...'.*

It is not surprising that interviewees who moved at later ages into schools where they did not already speak the language were more likely to have problems. The level and complexity of language needed by school children increases quite quickly year by year. Also by the age of 7, 8, 9 or 10, it is much more difficult for the children to not fall behind. It may take them up to a year to become able to understand most if not all of the content of the classes, and during this time, whilst they are still learning the language, they are missing out on the content of lessons that they do not understand. This content will be built on in future years, so missing out on it causes problems later on.

Shadi, Fatima and Mumtaz received language support in school and they all found it very helpful. Tom did not get any supplementary help. Some of the other interviewees had private tutors to help them make transitions between schools, even though in each case they already spoke the school language at home; however, Shadi, Tom, Fatima and Mumtaz did not have tutors, and nor did they attend Saturday supplementary schools. Nor in these four cases were parents available to work intensively with them (see Isabelle's account above). Despite this, both Tom and Shadi's experience shows that this can be done successfully, even though Tom and Shadi were in fact older than Fatima and Mumtaz when they moved, which might have led them to have more problems rather than less. To what extent did the fact that Fatima's parents had not attended school hold her back? How important was the whole year of school that she missed? Would Mumtaz's experience have been different if she had not missed so much school because of her mother's ill-health? Was it significant that Shadi already spoke three languages and Swedish was her fourth? Tom was already 'one of the better students' in his school in Croatia, so was this significant? It is not possible to definitively answer these questions, but below I extract some more general conclusions for parents who need to make decisions in the real world.

Generally, our interviewees found moving between schools easier when they already spoke the language used at their new school. Some had almost no issues at all, and where these did arise, they were often resolved relatively quickly. All of the interviewees could cope verbally in the classroom – they could understand, answer questions and participate. However, many had more problems with producing written work in their new school language. These varied from interviewees who were fluent orally but had to learn to read and write in that language from scratch, to those who were competent writers but perhaps needed some extra support. Some who had excelled in literature and writing in one language were frustrated that they could not achieve the same standard in a second language that they knew much less well. Even interviewees who did not change the language of schooling but changed countries still experienced some problems (new rules, different curriculums, the need to make friends and different ways of doing things), which reminds us that some of the issues attributed to language may actually be about culture, education systems or social norms and not about language at all.

- If your child will be starting school in a language that they do not understand or speak at the beginning of nursery and primary schooling (i.e. up to the age of around six), try to get them some exposure to this language in advance. This could be through attending a playgroup, meeting up with friends or neighbours, or through a childminder or mother's help. (Try to do so in ways that allow you to stick to your 'one person, one language' or 'one place, one language' approach or any other system that you have got going. Be careful not start to slide into using the majority language all the time. You may think that you are making a change temporarily to benefit your child, but it might be quite hard or impossible to change things back later on.) If you live somewhere with relatively flexible education authorities, you might be able to arrange for your child to start school a little early. You might also be able to enrol them in a private nursery using the same language. Depending on how much input they get, it is quite likely that your child will not actively speak the language as a result of this input, but the most important thing is that they are able to understand a little of what is going on. Starting school or nursery can be a little scary for some children, and, for these children, the fact that they may not understand much of what is happening around them may make the experience more frightening and make them feel even less in control.
- Make sure the school or nursery is aware of how much of the school's language medium the child knows.
- Do not worry if the school or nursery says your child is going through a silent phase. Children will often work out that there is no point speaking Arabic/Hungarian/Zulu to their new teacher, but they cannot yet manage to produce words or sentences in the school language. So they say nothing. This phase can last a few days or three months. It is quite normal and it just means that your child is absorbing the new language, and often they will start speaking it almost overnight when they feel ready to do so. Provided that your child speaks fluently for their age in your language, you should expect the possibility of a few teething problems but no long-term negative effects of starting school in a language they do not speak or understand.
- If a teacher or carer advises you that you should stop speaking your language to your child, please reread the section on changes as a result of advice given to parents (p.57) and the conclusions (pp.58–59). You may also want to consider whether this is the right school for your child because, if this teacher's views are representative, it is likely that the institution will be either ill informed about or hostile to bilingualism, or both.
- Parents planning to move children to a school where they do not already speak the language after the age of seven or eight should probably take steps to try to make the transition easier for their children, and should expect them to need more input and support to manage the change.
- If you have advanced warning of the move, try to arrange for your child to start to speak the school's medium language before the move.

- If the school does not offer additional support, see if you can arrange some language or study support out of school. You may be able to do this yourself. If you can find out what your children will be covering at school you can discuss the vocabulary for this with them at home in advance. If money is not a problem, you can, of course, pay a tutor. If this is not possible, you may be able to arrange some kind of swop with someone who can make use of a skill that you have or who wants to learn your language.
- As Tom notes, children who excel at maths or science may make the transition between schools using different languages more easily, but you can help with this by ensuring that they have all of the mathematical vocabulary they need in the new language as well as any different ways of doing things. (Be prepared for a child who excels at literacy to find this transition particularly hard, as the one thing that they are good at and probably enjoy most at school is turned upside down and may now be the thing that they have to struggle most with.)
- If your children are transitioning between schools in different countries, expect a certain degree of culture shock, even if the language remains the same. There will almost certainly be differences of curriculum as well as ways of doing things (e.g. maths) and quite possibly differences of dialect, idiom and in some cases spelling (US English rather than UK English for example).
- If your children are transitioning between schools in the same country or city using different languages, you should still probably expect a degree of culture shock and some time to adjust to differences in curriculum, teaching styles and methods.
- Do what you can to prepare your children for these transitions or support them through the process (by working with them at home, explaining why things are done differently etc.).
- You might be able to arrange for your children to spend time in a bilingual school which uses both languages, either long term or as a part of a transition process between two languages as Isabelle's family did.

15 Home Language Support/Teaching in Mainstream Schools

A few interviewees were offered support for their home language <u>as a home language</u> at school. All reported that this support was very positive. Far more of the interviewees attended classes where their home language was taught as a foreign language at school, which I discuss next. These experiences were very mixed, with at least as many interviews being negative about these classes as those who were positive. (Of course there were also many whose home language was never taught at any school.)

School Support for Home Languages

Only three interviewees were offered specific support for a language that they spoke at home. One was in 1940s Kenya, while the other two were more recent examples and both were in Sweden. One of the latter was Ingrid, who was offered weekly hour-long home language support classes after school. These classes were free and were organised by the school. Initially, lessons were one-to-one sessions with an English teacher. Later, when she was 15 or 16, she was taught in a group studying Shakespeare and other English literature. Ingrid was a child who refused to speak English at home and these lessons may have been important in helping her to maintain her active English between holidays. The classes were voluntary and Ingrid could have given them up but never felt that she wanted to.

Shadi told us that in Sweden the local authority was obliged to offer teaching in a child's home language at school. She was living in the north of Sweden and the school could not find a Farsi teacher and so they employed Shadi's mother (who had qualified as a teacher in Iran) to come and teach Farsi to her own children. The children finally sat both 'O' levels and 'A' levels in Farsi, and they did very well.

Parents raising children elsewhere – particularly in countries that are relatively affluent – may wonder whether similar provision could not be set up systematically in other countries.

The remaining example was Velji, who grew up speaking Gujarati at home, Swahili in the community and English at school in 1940s Kenya, which was then under British colonial rule. Velji attended a school especially for Asian boys in Mombasa. Here all the teaching was carried out in English. (This was prior to independence when Swahili was introduced as a major language medium in Kenyan schools.) At school, the boys also had tuition in their home language (either Hindi, Urdu or Gujarati), and this was where Velji learnt to read and write in Gujarati. His family had books in Gujarati at home and both his parents were literate in Gujarati. This system was segregated and inegalitarian, but in terms of the support for the boys' home languages, was nonetheless very progressive.

Home Languages Taught as a Foreign Language at School

This was a much larger group – 14 interviewees – with very mixed experiences. Some interviewees had choices about which foreign languages they could take, others did not. Many interviewees and their parents saw these classes as an opportunity for children speaking a language at home to improve their written skills, their grammar or their spelling. Others felt that these classes were a waste of time for children who were already fluent speakers of a language. Some teachers welcomed these children into the class as a valuable resource and made use of them, whereas others clearly felt threatened and worried that these children would notice mistakes in the teacher's own command of the language in question (sadly, in some cases with good reason). Several interviewees were excluded from these classes and were given different reasons for this – including some very unhelpful ones. Clearly most, if not all, of the interviewees found the lessons very easy and did very well in them – however, some felt that expectations of them were very high, and that they were expected to be perfect. Some prioritised their work in other subjects as they felt that they did not need to study in this area, and thus did not do so well. Some brought their knowledge from home to school, and this was welcomed by the teachers. Others did so and were rebuffed or corrected in ways that now seem unhelpful – and are clearly remembered by and still emotionally resonate with the interviewees today.

I start with some of the more positive experiences. Claudia viewed her beginners' English lessons positively, although she had otherwise spent much of her education in either English-medium schools or in international schools. In Germany, when she was attending an ordinary state school and was in the standard English class for beginners, she says, unsurprisingly, that, *'I was always the best in the class'*. But she says that she did not mind studying this basic level even though she was a fluent speaker. Similarly, Markus 'learnt' English at school in Germany and obviously found his English lessons very easy. He took A-levels in English when finishing school in Germany. Despite his knowledge of English he did not find English lessons boring, but instead found them rather interesting: *'... actually I learnt a few things; it's quite good to learn the basics. I didn't resent that I had to sit there ...'.*

We now turn to those whose experiences were more mixed or ambiguous, and finally some that are discouraging or even shocking.

Many interviewees found the lessons boring but still feel that they gained something from them. Christine was one interviewee who spoke German already but studied German as a foreign language together with her class. Not surprisingly, she was top of the class. She says that the classes were boring. Her first teacher taught extremely slowly. This was not just Christine's natural frustration as she was already pretty fluent, as she discovered when she moved school after two years and found that her old class was way behind in the syllabus and her new class several terms ahead. Christine said that she rarely learnt any grammar rules in her German classes – she would just ask herself what sounded right – as a native speaker can and does. However, the classes did teach her to read and write in German, which she had not learnt at home (you may remember that Christine's mother had been advised to stop speaking German with her children and so Christine's German was maintained almost entirely through visits to family in Germany – see p.57). One problem with her German classes was that the teacher was, of course, teaching High German, and Christine mainly knew her mother's dialect. At first, Christine thought that the teacher was speaking funny or pronouncing things wrong. But she did get used to this and her teachers corrected her pronunciation and some grammatical differences, so that Christine can now speak fluently in both High German and the Baadische dialect.

Armelle's case is interesting as she is trilingual, and was taught two languages as foreign languages with different experiences. Armelle had grown up in a mixed-language family speaking French and Spanish, but the family also moved to Italy for her father's work for seven years, where she learnt Italian from the community and the TV although she attended the international French school. It was here that she first learnt English as a foreign language at school – at 14 she needed to add a new language and had the choice between German and Spanish. *'My father wanted to me to take German, but my mother wanted me to take Spanish, so that if we went back to Argentina I would have all of the perfect grammar so I did three years of basic Spanish'.*

Thus, Armelle went into a class of Spanish for beginners, but she found this very boring and got into trouble when she read books in class. She would help complete other students' homework and help them do tests. The teacher would ask her to help (despite her Argentinean accent). She would ask Armelle to read out texts to the class and would point out the differences in accents. This older and stricter teacher gave Armelle the same very basic work that all the class were doing – possibly because the French system is quite rigid. Despite Armelle's mother's hope that these lessons would help Armelle's grammar, she does not feel that they helped at all with her grammar or written Spanish – in fact, she had already reached a high-level and the classes were just too basic. Armelle also studied Italian as a fourth language and here she did feel that these lessons helped improve her grammar. Her written Italian was not as good as her written Spanish, but it may also have helped that this teacher, who she describes as 'young and cool', did set Armelle different and more advanced work.

In contrast to Armelle, in (German and English-speaking) Sarah's case it was decided that she should not learn German at school as her mother felt the standard of German teaching was not that good, so she decided to learn Spanish instead. There was some discussion about this at the time, as Sarah wanted to learn to read and write properly in German and would have opted to do the German classes if the choice had been left up to her.

Like Armelle, Daniela's French teacher also wanted to use her as a resource in her French classes, but, unlike Armelle, Daniela did not appreciate this and she did not cooperate. Her teacher was *'really excited about this French student coming into the school, and she really wanted me to be the teacher's pet, and I am not that kind of person…and she was so desperate to have this perfect French student. I was not going to be a teacher's pet! Subsequently, I was very naughty in her French class!'* French was a compulsory subject and Daniela was very bored during the lessons; she did not want to work hard in French because she did not want to be the perfect pet for her teacher so other kids would not turn against her. *'I didn't want to be that person who really stood out!'*

Other interviewees felt that they should have been used as a resource in these classes or at least should have been included but were not. Despite Ingrid's positive experience of home language support in Sweden where she had one hour's English tuition a week, when her classmates started to learn English Ingrid was not allowed to participate in the classes and was sent away into another room where she had to listen to audio tapes in Swedish. This was not a positive experience – at the time, she wondered whether the teacher felt that her Swedish was not good and hence felt that she needed the extra input in Swedish, which knocked her confidence somewhat. Now she wonders if the teacher just thought that the basic English lessons would be a waste of her time. Ironically, Ingrid does feel that she may have missed out on some of the basic English grammar and spelling. *'I have learned English through speaking it, the way children learn it. But when you go to school you learn grammar and spelling and all that. … I do feel that I haven't really received the basic grammar and spelling. … I still feel that I could have picked up a bit more basic grammar'.* Ingrid also remembers being told a couple of times by teachers: *'Well you speak two languages ok but not one perfectly',* and she recalls that she had *'(British) English teachers who corrected me for spelling words the correct American way. Things like that have affected me and I did wonder whether I did just speak two languages superficially'.*

In Christopher's case, he was the only French-speaking pupil in the English school where French was taught as a foreign language. During the French lessons his teacher used to tell him: *'You know French, just go to the back of the class and do what you like'.* Now, in retrospect, Christopher thinks he could have been used as a resource in the classroom, *'He could have asked me to speak French to other people, perhaps. The lessons were very boring. … When I took French O-level, I got an A without any work'.*

Sylvia was the only English-speaking pupil in her French school. She remembers being sent out of beginners' English classes for being cheeky, and despite some attempts to find ways to use her as a resource for the other children, it was eventually agreed that she would go to the library and do homework during these classes. She feels that the teachers did not like having a child in the class who had a better accent and pronunciation than them, and that this was part of the reason why the issue was solved in this way. That said, it seemed that being allowed to skip these classes was a privilege and not a punishment. After one year, children were able to choose between English and German as a foreign language, and so Sylvia joined the German class.

Helen (whose father spoke English to her at home in Holland) attended English foreign language classes in both primary and secondary school. In secondary school, she found the classes easy but she found that there were aspects of the language that she did not know including grammar and areas of vocabulary, and so she did not feel that this was a waste of time. She did feel that she was expected to have perfect English, which was something she did not have – in fact she would usually prioritise her other homework knowing that she could get a reasonable mark in English without working very hard. Hence she felt that expectations on her were very high and hard to live up to. Helen was also one of the interviewees who brought language that they had learnt at home to school, but this prompted negative reactions. She particularly remembers one occasion when she had a test and had to give a meaning for a word – she had not revised and gave her own definition of the word (which was correct), but she was reprimanded by the teacher because she had used her own words and not the definition in the book.

Isabelle probably had the worst experience in a foreign language class. When in France she needed to sit through a beginner's level English class which she would have found boring and frustrating anyway, but it was made even worse by the fact that the English teacher regularly: ' ... *made mistakes – for example, she would write "sandwich" with an "sh" at the end. And I'd be like "that's wrong". She hated me. She had it in for me. She'd send me out to sit in the hall. She apparently told the other children in the class that I couldn't speak English properly. I understand now why she hated me but it was horrible. It made me angry'.*

Like Christopher, several of the interviewees sat exams in their home language without any tuition or at least without having to work. Isabelle again (this time back in the United States) had little or no input in French for two years during the last two years of high school. She did an advanced placement system, which included an exam in French. She did not attend the classes but was given the reading list one week before the exam, read the books and got the top mark.

Saadia did one year of classes at school in Urdu, but this was a mixed experience. She found that she was able to write very neatly in Urdu and of course she could understand and talk quite fluently which seemed to lead the teacher to believe that she was far more literate in Urdu than was actually the case. This meant that Saadia was asked to do more advanced things – which she did not feel competent or capable of.

Conclusion

These varying experiences involve a large number of variables: the interviewees' fluency in the language they were taught, teachers' different personalities and differences in the style and systems of education, as well as differences of personality between the interviewees. This is an area in which parents need to feel their way carefully. One would hope that many schools now would handle these issues better – although several of the negative experiences came from interviewees who are relatively young, so these experiences are sadly quite recent. The fact that so many of the interviewees did have mixed or negative experiences at one time or another suggests that this is an area that parents should watch closely and be ready to intervene if they feel that things may be going wrong.

- I am not aware that formal support for all home languages is routinely available anywhere except in Sweden, and I hear that it is in decline and may not even continue to be offered there. (There is much more support for some 'national' languages, e.g. Welsh in Wales, French in northern Italy etc.) Parents elsewhere may want to lobby for this because it does seem extremely useful, both symbolically and practically.

- You may have no choice at all, but many families do have choices. Some opt for a child taking the relatively easy option of 'learning' a language that they in fact already know – filling in some gaps, consolidating what they have, and having at least one class at school in which they can excel, be the best in the class and not have to work too hard to succeed. If your child is finding other subjects or aspects of their life difficult or has little free time, you may be more likely to go for this approach. The downsides are that they may be bored, their knowledge may challenge the teacher and they may not behave well. You might be able to find out if the school/teacher would be willing to set different and more advanced work for your child, as one of Armelle's teachers did.

- However, do not expect your child's language to be perfect. And make sure that your child knows that he or she may need to study if they want to do well – just as in any other subject. Although it is true that some children did extremely well in exams without any work at all, this was not true for all children.

- Some children who already spoke a language still felt that they did benefit from strengthening their reading and writing in a language and consolidating basic grammar.

- For some children who had either never had input in a language at home (Astrid) or for whom this had ceased (Christine), foreign language classes were a significant factor allowing children to continue to maintain and even develop their languages, although I would not count on this as an ideal strategy.

- At school, children will normally learn a standard received pronunciation and grammar, which may be helpful in a context where there are dialects and regional accents. If this is the case for you, you might want to explain to your child that the teacher will teach, for example, 'German as it is spoken in Berlin, not as it is spoken in the village where Grandma lives', so that they are forewarned that it may sound different and use different forms.

- The other option is that the children learn a completely new language from scratch. As there is some evidence that multilingual people find it easier to learn additional languages, this may also be a very positive option. And if your children are finding school relatively easy and need a new challenge, or if you are concerned about your child being bored or misbehaving in a class that is too easy, you may opt for this approach.

- Where only one language is on offer and it is the one that your children already speak and understand, there may still be options if you and your school are prepared to be just a little flexible or creative. One primary school we are aware of in London, which was arranging for groups of children to be taught basic French, arranged for a group of around a dozen children who spoke French at home to have a separate lesson during the lunch hour, which was geared to their level so that they did not attend the very basic sessions with their classmates. (This was only possible as the children were attending the French classes in groups of 15 and not whole classes. The only extra cost to the school was half an hour of the teacher's time.)

- If your child is going to 'learn' a language alongside beginner classmates, try to make sure that the school and the individual teacher is fully aware of how well your child speaks, reads and writes a language that they will be taught at school. Try to have a conversation with the foreign language teaching staff who will be teaching your child. This may allow you to assess their attitude and level of confidence in their own competence in the language in question. Depending on your child's character and your conclusions from meeting and talking with the teacher, decide if your child might be set more advanced work, used as a resource in the class for other children or could get on with some other work – either homework or additional work that could be set and marked by you during these lessons.

- If you and the school agree that your child will not attend these classes, make sure that your child is given very positive reasons for this and is not left to conclude, as Ingrid did, that this is because they are deficient in some other way.

16 Additional Support Outside (or as an alternative to) Mainstream Schools

We also asked interviewees what their experiences had been of other forms of support and input in their languages organised outside mainstream schools. This was primarily Saturday or supplementary schools. One interviewee also had some experience of home education. In this section we also discuss what interviewees recollected about the process of learning to read and write in several languages.

Saturday Schools

In many areas in the UK, parents have got together to organise self-funding supplementary schools that take place either one day in the week after school, or on Saturdays. Schools have different priorities but generally teach reading and writing in a home language, most also support verbal language skills and many help pass on the wider culture and heritage associated with a language. Many parents feel that, in addition to the actual tuition given, such schools can be useful in giving children a peer group of other children who speak a language. This often helps with the issue of children feeling that they do not fit in. There were six interviewees who had attended such schools, which are probably more common now than they were over two decades ago. (There was only one example of a supplementary school outside of the UK, and that was in Australia.)

Once again our interviewees, though, had very different and very mixed experiences at these schools. I will start with the most positive experiences.

Astrid grew up in Australia, the child of two German parents. Astrid's parents decided not to speak German to her at home and, apart from a six-month stay in Germany when she was four years old, a Saturday German language school was her primary input in German. Astrid started Saturday school when she was between seven and eight years old, and attended until she was 10. *'We were immersed in German. It was the main purpose of being there. It was very strict, typical German'*. Despite this strictness, Astrid enjoyed going to the Saturday school. *'Everyone had one focus there, to learn German. We all had German parents and we had similar interests. It was quite nice to be with people in the same situation'*. Although Astrid was not so wholeheartedly positive at the time, it was a *'Very positive experience when I look at it now! At the time, of course, friends were playing out on a Saturday and me going to a German school! I think it's a great concept. Fantastic concept. We used to sing choir songs, just the intensity of learning the language. Everything is in German, you speak in German, you have good books to read in German, it was quite a novelty I thought, unusual thing to do'.* Although she describes the school as strict, Astrid also found it enjoyable. *'There was an element of fun, the choir. I always enjoyed learning, I found it advanced'.* Astrid did not tell all her friends at regular school about her Saturday school. *'My friends at school didn't know I was going to a German school! You know kids…'.* As she was a good athlete she wanted to do sport at weekends and stopped going to German classes when she was 10 years old. Her father was very supportive of her athletics and this was a mutual decision with her parents. After this, Astrid's only input in German was in her German as a foreign language classes in mainstream school until she studied German at university. However, she considers herself bilingual and speaks German fluently today.

Susanne was similarly positive about the German language Saturday school in the UK, which was set up and initially run by her mother (who was a teacher). The school was linked to the German church where her father was the pastor. Susanne saw it as an opportunity for German language and culture to be presented as acceptable, although sometimes she also thought that the content was too simple and could be boring. When she was 15, Susanne became a teacher at the school and she continued to teach there for about two to three years until she went to university.

However, for most of our interviewees, these schools were not particularly valued by the children whilst they were attending, although many interviewees had changed their minds about this as adults. In general, it was difficult for children to have to study an extra day when they would rather be out playing. But there were also some other more specific issues that interviewees raised about their time at such schools.

Antony (growing up speaking Greek at home in London) raises two issues that correspond to the experience of children I am aware of through the Waltham Forest Bilingual Group. The first is that the style of teaching in these schools was often much more formal and less participatory or interactive than the style that most children in the UK now experience in mainstream primary schools. So Antony felt that the Greek schoolteachers were pushy, and that the school used a different method of teaching compared to the English system that seemed to him more social and interactive. Greek was taught in completely different way where the teachers tried to teach as much as they could during a limited time. As a consequence, Antony found the English system much more enjoyable. This type of contrast can lead to children being less willing to attend Saturday schools.

The second issue that Antony had with the Greek school that he attended was that he started there relatively late (when he was seven or eight years old). In his English primary school, despite having started school with no English, Antony was doing pretty well at the English curriculum. However, not surprisingly, having started later than many of the other pupils and having never learnt to read or write in Greek, he found that he was struggling at the Greek school. He felt demotivated because he was behind instead of being ahead of others in the class. Altogether, Antony sums up his experience of the Greek school as a painful exercise and he says that he hated it.

Vera W did not attend a Chinese school until she was 10 years old. As her family lived outside London, this meant getting up early and getting the train into London with her sister who also attended. Unlike Antony, Vera W had been taught to read and write in Chinese at home by her mother and then by a cousin. Nonetheless, she says that, *'I remember resenting having to do the Chinese homework. You had to do a lot of repetitions [copying out Chinese characters lots of times]. I remember my hand really aching and I didn't want to go anymore. I was the oldest child attending the school – many of the children attending had been born in China or Hong Kong and had gone to school in China'.* She remembers that the school was strict – if you did not do all of the homework you would get told off. She did not know any of the other children. She does not remember any other activities at the school, like songs, drama, music, craft or other activities linked to cultural festivals, although she knows that there are schools that exist now with a much wider set of activities. She went for about six months to a year, which she now feels was not long enough, and she wishes that her mother had encouraged or pushed her to continue going for longer.

Although Saadia's experience of a community school was not negative, she dropped out after a couple of years: Saadia started to go to an Urdu Saturday school when she was six or seven, but she dropped out after one or two years. She thinks that this may have been because of her mother's work schedule and her family commitments. Saadia does not remember that she said anything about this or, at the time, asked if she could continue to go, although she now regrets not continuing in the school.

In Bindi's case, when the family came to England, there were no Gujarati schools in existence. A Gujarati school started when Bindi was 14, and although Bindi's mother may have suggested that she and her sister attend, there was not any pressure or compulsion from her parents that they should do so, but she and her sister decided to go along and they continued for one summer. However, Bindi and her sister were the oldest children by far, whereas most of the others were 5, 6 or 7 years old and they were all studying at the same level. Bindi and her sister felt very awkward about this and, coupled with the fact that they were studying for their 'O' levels, decided that they should concentrate on that and the Gujarati school was dropped.

Mohammed had the most negative experience of a Saturday or community school: from the age of 8 to 12, he attended a Bengali Saturday morning school where he learnt to read in Bengali. He did not attend the school willingly and had to be made to go. He preferred watching TV. He would also play truant from this school (which he never did from his junior school). The teacher at the school used corporal punishment on the children who were naughty (including Mohammed), and Mohammed could not accept this. Finally, on one occasion when he was beaten, he retaliated and (clearly to his relief) he was expelled.

Home Education

Although I have described some examples of parents and other relatives supporting their children at particular times above, no interviewee in our sample was educated at home as an alternative to mainstream schools. Home schooling is probably more common now than it was over two decades ago, and we are aware of bilingual families that are currently educating their children at home in London. However, one family in our sample essentially duplicated their children's education so that they went to mainstream school and then studied again at home in Farsi. Whilst her family migrated around Europe, living in France, the UK and finally Sweden, Shadi explained that her mother, who had qualified as a teacher in Iran before they had had to leave, *'taught us, rigidly, the whole of the first primary school curriculum in Farsi. You know literature, history, geography, maths, science …. She had all of the books. … She did it in the evenings and weekends, particularly in the school holidays. I remember in the summer holidays we used to have to study for at least three hours a day when all of our friends were playing outside. She was very strict. We had to sit exams and if we didn't pass the exams we had to study for a month and sit another exam at the end of the holidays. My brother and I both sat the official Iranian exams and passed with full marks and now I am very grateful'.*

Biliteracy – Reading and Writing in Two Languages

More than half of our interviewees, in the end, somehow learnt to read and write in both or all their languages – some as adults through evening classes and so on. For some children this involved learning several different alphabets, different writing systems, learning that some languages are written from right to left and some from left to right. However, very few reported any long-term difficulty in doing this. Some interviewees were in bilingual schools or alternately moved between schools using different languages, and thus they could hardly avoid learning to read and write in both languages. However, this was not always totally painless (see Matilde's account of learning to read and write in French aged 11, despite her already good spoken French on p.116). Some interviewees were taught to read at home by their parents before starting school so, for example, in France children are taught to read at around six years old and Sylvia's mother taught her children to read in English at home before they were taught at school. Some developed these written skills in their home language through being taught the language as a foreign language.

Many interviewees where both or all the languages they spoke used the same script transferred the skills from one language across to the other without much or any help. Helen learnt to read in Dutch at school in Holland. She transferred from this into being able to read English without any formal learning, although she rarely read in English for pleasure as a child. Camilla remembers having Danish books, which she loved, although no one particularly taught her to read in Danish and she also transferred the skills over from having learnt to read and write in English at school. However, others found that even when reading using the same scripts, their biliteracy remained very limited without any additional input. Pedro lived in bilingual but segregated Texas, speaking Spanish and English. His family had some books around at home which Pedro had used to teach himself to read, but these were all in English and, although he could transfer some skills across, he was not confident in reading in Spanish until he got to high school and had the opportunity to study Spanish formally. Despite talking a mixture of Spanish and English with his family at home, when he later moved away and wrote letters home he always did so exclusively in English. Pedro lived in a community where Spanish was generally not valued. This was even more the case with Occitan in south-western France where Sophie lived. Occitan was a language that had rarely ever been written down, but Sophie was very fortunate to have an uncle who had written poetry and some books in Occitan that had been published. Sophie was thus very unusually able to learn to read in Occitan, because they had some of the original typed transcripts of these books in the house. When she could already read in French, she remembers sitting down with her grandfather and working through them together – she remembers that her grandfather had some difficulty in working out what was written down in Occitan too. As far as she is aware, neither of her parents had learned to read in Occitan.

Although most of these accounts make the process sound very easy (at least where the same alphabets are being used), we must not forget Marion, whose father had started to teach her to read and write in Welsh at the same time, or just before she started to learn to read and write in English at school. Marion seems to have resisted learning to read or write in either language until the family moved to Cardiff when she was 10, where she had a teacher who spoke Welsh – within a year, she was reading heavy texts full of complex language in English (for more details, see p.111).

Interviewees whose languages used different scripts needed more input in order to learn to read and write in a language that they were not schooled in. Mohammed learned Bengali at his Saturday school. Vera W remembers being taught to read and write in Chinese by one of her cousins, who was very good at calligraphy. She remembers when she was taught to write numbers in Chinese how much easier the numbers were to write than in English. Otherwise, although she could read in both languages, she does not remember noticing the different writing and reading systems or trying to apply one system to the other language. As described above (p.132), Vera W went on to attend the Chinese Saturday school for a short period.

Shadi learnt to read both English and Farsi at the same time. The two languages use different alphabets and one is written left to right and one right to left. She was taught to read and write by her mother at home and said: *'I was never confused because the writing systems are so different. I don't remember finding it very difficult'*.

Antony learnt to read and write Greek at the Saturday school, which, as described above, he hated. He spoke Greek first and then English, but as far as reading and writing were concerned this was the opposite. He found reading in English easy due to his visual memory, and although he transferred these skills into the Greek alphabet he found it difficult to master the accents, which are key to understanding in Greek but which are not used in English.

There were also nine interviewees who never learnt to read or write in one of their languages as children. Most of these regretted this. Five either opted to take an evening class or taught themselves to read and write as adults. In Saad's case, he never studied in Kurdish or learnt Kurdish at school; the only second language taught at Saad's school in Iraq was English. Although Saad's father could read and write in Kurdish, he did not teach his children to do so. Saad has taught himself to read and write Kurdish as an adult. He feels that he has reached a good level in reading, but feels he still needs to work more on his writing. The Kurdish used in Iraqi Kurdistan is written in Arabic script and uses the same letters, with just one or two additional letters to represent sounds that do not exist in Arabic. This meant that it was relatively easy for Saad to transfer the reading and writing skills he had from Arabic to Kurdish. However, despite the fact that all the verbal interactions within the family were in Kurdish (Saad's family were the most consistent family of all on this point, see p.66), Saad wrote a lot of letters to his family home in Baghdad from England after he left Iraq, but all of these letters were written in Arabic.

Fatima, aged 17, went to an adult education centre to formally study Arabic which she had not done since she left Morocco, and she sat and passed the exam at the end of the course which was something that she felt that she needed to do. Sabina completed university and then she decided to study Urdu at an evening class and gained an 'O'-level qualification. At around this time, she also made a conscious decision that she would speak Urdu to her father because she really wanted to maintain and improve her Urdu. Despite this effort, she is still not very confident in reading and writing in Urdu and says that although she can and does read children's books to her son, she would not read an adult novel in Urdu. She comments on this: *'That's the downside of not being able to read a language; that you can't improve your vocabulary ...'.* But on the plus side, the fact that she can read and write some Urdu has helped, *'In Urdu there are different "R" sounds and I may get a sound wrong, but if I can see [a word] written down, I do know which "R" to use'.*

When Parvati was at university, she learnt to speak, read and write Sanskrit (which is related to Hindi in a similar way in which Latin is related to modern-day Italian) but she has never learnt to read or write Hindi per se. She said that as the languages are related, learning Sanskrit reinforced her vocabulary in particular, and as a result of having learnt Sanskrit she quite often surprises her older relatives by knowing a word in Hindi that they (momentarily) cannot remember.

Many of Velji's experiences have been unusual or different, and this is also true of his experience of learning to write a language relatively late in life. He was raised in Kenya speaking Gujarati at home, English at school and Swahili on the street. By the age of 16 Velji could speak fluently in several dialects of Gujarati, as well as English and Swahili, and he could read and write in English and Gujarati, but not in Swahili. For many years, part of his job involved travelling along the coast of Kenya and Tanzania checking on the sales of British American Tobacco (BAT) products. This enabled him to learn other dialects of both Swahili and Gujarati. He also taught himself to read Swahili during this time – he explains that Swahili is written in roman script and so he found it relatively easy to read letters from his Swahili-speaking suppliers and so on. He retired from BAT relatively early and decided to live in the UK. He did not want to stop working completely, and it was suggested to him that he could build a new career out of his strong and unusual language skills. He decided to train as an interpreter. At this time, he also studied Swahili formally so that he could be confident writing Swahili. Up to this point, as he was self-taught, he was not confident that he could write without making mistakes.

Four interviewees still do not read or write in at least one of their languages today. One did not comment at all on this issue; two regretted it, and only one did not. Pari did not attend a Saturday school and never learned to read Gujarati. She does not regret this as she feels that reading and writing was not essential for her Gujarati interactions within the family, although, for her, speaking Gujarati certainly was essential.

In contrast, Bindi (who happens to be Velji's daughter), said: *'As an adult, I became very aware that it was very important to be multilingual. And I had these regrets about not learning to read and write in Gujarati … as I became a young adult I often told my Mum "Why didn't you teach us to read and write?" And to this day I regret it, because even though I wouldn't use it on a daily basis, through the [written] language you learn the culture much more deeply and I believe that very strongly. I think that you understand a culture from a much deeper perspective if you can read that language too. Now I just don't have the time, [to learn] and I feel that it was a missed opportunity'.*

Saadia also said she regretted *'the fact that I didn't keep going to Saturday school. I wish that I had learnt much more and I wish that I was much more confident in Urdu especially reading and writing. I wish I had also learnt to read Punjabi. I could have done GCSE Urdu … Sometimes I wonder if we should go and live in Pakistan, but the fact that I don't read and write in Urdu would make this difficult'.*

Conclusion

There is no doubt that many children do find Saturday school rewarding and enjoyable and benefit from having a peer group there. Even though Saturday schools were not always popular with interviewees when they were children – and many of the schools had very real faults or limitations – all of interviewees appreciated what they had gained through attending their schools once they were adults. It is certainly worth going out of your way to find or to set up a Saturday school or a similar group where your children can learn different facets of a minority language. And if this is not possible for you, consider whether you can teach your children at home or arrange for someone else to do so.

All of our interviewees who could read and write in both or all of their languages were very grateful that they were able to do so. Those interviewees who had not learnt to read and write as children often went to some trouble to learn to do so as adults by attending evening classes or teaching themselves. All but one of the four interviewees who had never learnt to read or write in one of their languages regretted this. Several interviewees mentioned the wider benefits of being able to read in terms of access to culture and a deeper knowledge of the language.

- One clear suggestion for parents from these experiences is to try to ensure that children start a supplementary school as early as possible. If there is no existing school near where you live, but there is a group of multilingual families speaking your language, it is relatively easy to set up a small Saturday school or group, and you do not need to be formally trained as a teacher to organise activities for primary age children. If you do join late, your child may feel that they are already very behind when they see younger children work at the same level or ahead, and this may be demotivating for them.

- If finding or setting up a school is not possible, parents who are themselves literate in the home language can replicate many of the activities that would normally be run at a supplementary school at home with their children (as many of our children's parents did, e.g. Sylvia in France who learnt to read from her mother in English). If, at a later time, these children have an opportunity to attend a supplementary school, they will not need to start at the beginning with classes of very young children. The internet offers a lot of resources now in many languages, as well as the possibility of families meeting and talking virtually using webcams and, with a little creativity, this may make it possible to create a virtual school or language group. Some suggested places that you can look for advice or support in setting up a school or teaching children from home are listed in the references section of this book on p. 225. (Of course working from home will not give your child a peer group – except possibly a virtual one – in the same way as a school that meets physically.)

- Parents who have a choice of schools may want to try to choose one that has a teaching style which is similar to that the children experience at primary school. Others may decide that a particular style of teaching is culturally appropriate (perhaps because the parents will have experienced that teaching style themselves as children). In this case, it may be worth explaining in some detail why this style is more appropriate and why it is different, as this may help children to accept the differences in educational styles and, in particular, not react negatively to a Saturday school that is stricter or more formal than a school the child attends during the week.

- Almost without exception, the interviewees referred to the fact that as children they did not appreciate having to attend these classes. They referred to the things that they would prefer to be doing on a Saturday. However, every interviewee who did attend such classes was very grateful that they had done so once they were adults. Equally, those who did not continue to attend classes, with only one exception, wished that they had gone for longer and/or that their parents had insisted that they attend. Apart from Mohammed, all of those who dropped out regretted this later.

- If your child's two or more languages use the same script, they may be able to transfer reading skills from one language to another with little or no external help.

- Even if the script is identical, however, unless your language is particularly phonetic (i.e. written down exactly as it sounds), children will need more help and support to be able to learn to write using the correct grammar and spelling.

- No child reported confusion or difficulty learning to read and write using two scripts or writing systems. If this is your situation, our advice to parents would be to treat reading and writing in exactly the same way as speaking (i.e. to teach it to children in parallel at the same time, and not wait until a child has mastered one language before teaching a second). The only child who reported any difficulty or confusion about reading and writing in two languages was Marion – and in any event, her two languages (English and Welsh) use the same alphabet. (For more on this, see also Charmian Kenner's excellent book in the bibliography.)
- Interviewees with limited literacy skills find that it limits their access to culture and means that they do not extend or add to their vocabulary.
- Interviewees who did not learn to read and write in their languages as children typically went on to learn to do so as adults, and so clearly were very motivated to take on the extra work that this involved.

17 Help with Homework

Another dilemma that often causes concern to parents – but also one that tends to creep up on people so that a habit has been established without any conscious decision being taken – concerns which language you use whilst you are helping a child with their homework. So we asked in our interviews what parents had done and how the interviewees had found this. Quite a large proportion of our interviewees said that they had never had help with their homework. In some cases, interviewees were bright and did not ask for any help. For others, it seems that it was simply not the done thing in their culture for parents to help their children with homework. In other cases, the fact that the homework was in a language that neither parent was confident reading and writing was a factor. This applied to some of the children of migrants, as well as to some of the children who were learning an additional language purely through school. Parents who had quite a limited knowledge of the language used at school could still help children when they were very young. So Mumtaz remembers that when she was given English words to take home and learn every day, she would read them with her father: *'He would help me and he would praise me'*. This was despite the fact that Mumtaz's father's written English was not very good – and this is still the case, as she continues to help him fill in forms today.

Other parents helped with specific tasks in a language that was not their mother tongue. The French educational system requires children to learn all the different forms of irregular verbs by heart, and several parents who spoke another language to their children still spent considerable time drilling their children on these conjugations in French. Sylvia and Armelle both recalled their mothers who more usually spoke to them in English and Spanish respectively doing this in France.

As the interviewees got older though, and the homework became more complex, parents that were not fluent in a language were often no longer able to help. We mentioned above (see p.54) that Ingrid noticed this most acutely because of a very sharp contrast when her Swedish father died when she was 11 years old. After her father's death Ingrid did not have anyone who could read and check her essays or homework and point out any errors before it was handed in.

In some families, the interviewees' older brothers or sisters provided this support if it was needed. So Velji, who studied in English and spoke Gujarati at home with his family, remembers getting occasional help with homework from his elder brothers who also went to the English-medium school. For some interviewees help was available for some subjects but not others. While Snjezana was attending the Italian language school in Croatia (and was the only Italian speaker in the family) she could not get help with a lot of her work, but she remembers her sister helping her with her science homework in Croatian, although Snjezana herself was working in Italian and the work to be handed in was in that language. In her migrant family, Shadi also said that her father would help with her homework if it was science or maths, but no one at home could help her with literature or with writing in English or Swedish – in fact, Shadi would help her father if he had to do a piece of writing in English or Swedish.

However, even help with maths was not guaranteed. Another interviewee, Sylvia, said that her mother had some difficulties helping her with maths homework, as the French used a different system to do the sums. To this day, for Sylvia, despite the fact that in most other areas her English is now probably her dominant language, numbers are in French and if she has difficulties remembering a phone number, she will say it in French rather than English, which will help her to recall it.

Where parents spoke both the school language and a different home language, the families had a choice about whether to use the former or the latter to do homework. Some parents feel that their children will be disadvantaged at school if they do not get help with homework in the school language. Others feel that using the school language will dilute the rule that only the home language is spoken at home, which will mean that the school and majority language is used more and more at home to the detriment of the minority language. The two families that had the clearest and most consistent rules about language use at home also applied this to homework. In Saad's case, all homework support was in Kurdish – the minority language – and not Arabic, his school language. So Saad would bring work home to be completed in Arabic and his father would help him with it, but his father would speak only Kurdish to Saad when he did so. Similarly: *'Even when [my father and older siblings] taught me English, it was in Kurdish'*. Saad explains that, for his English homework, his family would do the instructions and explanations in Kurdish and then use some English words as needed. Any translation of a word he did not understand in English would be into Kurdish rather than Arabic.

Sylvia's mother was a bit more relaxed, but she still used English to help her children with their homework. Sylvia remembers that a lot of homework had to be done in French – such as reading aloud from a French reading book, and French verbs that had to be learnt off by heart in different forms. Her mother would help her with these in French. On other occasions her mother might read a French text in a book and then discuss it with her children in English. Vera W also remembers her mother helping her to do her English homework, although she would speak in Cantonese when she did so.

But for many other families, as mentioned above (see p.70), talking about school topics or helping with homework was also a moment when the majority and school language entered households that had until then operated a 'one place, one language' rule, or which interfered with a 'one person, one language' rule.

Conclusion

- Some interviewees, like Ingrid, did feel that they missed out a little if they did not have a fluent speaker of the school language at home to help with homework, but not all did so. Many parents did help younger children effectively with a language that they were really not at all fluent in. And it is worth remembering that Ingrid's recollection of deep embarrassment, which still affects her mildly today, came at a time when she had just been bereaved and must have been feeling particularly vulnerable.

- For homework tasks that are very language dependent (writing stories, or essays, comprehension or grammar exercises), if you are in this position, and if you feel that your child might lack confidence or would welcome some extra support, you might want to see if you could ask a sibling, other relatives, a neighbour or a friend who is fluent in the school language if they would mind helping out either regularly or just from time to time if a piece of work was particularly difficult or important.

- For homework tasks that are not language dependent, you should just help your child in your language, as Snjezana's sister and Shadi's father usefully did.

- For families where one or both of the parents normally speak a minority language at home, but are also competent speakers of the school language, you will need to make a choice. As described above, there are some tasks that will perhaps require some use of the school language (e.g. learning spellings or conjugating verbs, writing essays, and comprehension or grammar exercises). For everything else, the more ambitious choice, at least from the point of view of bringing up children multilingually, is to help the children with homework in the home/minority language. This has several key advantages. It will help maintain and extend the children's vocabulary in the home language, it can help maintain a clear division or rule about language use at home, and experts also argue that a child may well have a deeper, more complete and more robust understanding of a topic if it has been discussed with them separately in two different languages. Still, many parents do seem to feel intuitively that helping in the language of the school for other less language dependent tasks such as maths, science or history will lead to a better outcome in terms of the children's progress at school, but there is not a lot of evidence that this is the case and the reverse may well be true. On the downside, help with homework in a home language may well take a bit longer because the children absorb the terms needed in that language if they are not already familiar with them, and you may well encounter more resistance from the children if you do it this way. Thus once again, we come down to a personal decision about what feels most right for your family based on the parent's and children's competence in their various languages, and the amount of time that parents have available.

- Be aware that systems for doing even basic maths calculations vary widely between countries. If you teach the child the system that you were taught, this might be a little confusing for them (and for their teacher).

- As mentioned above, this is an issue that can creep up on families who fall into habits with no conscious decision ever being taken, as the child(ren) begin bringing home very limited homework but this gradually builds up over the years. If you do decide to routinely help children in the school and not a home language, try to set limits to this so that this is not the beginning of a process of attrition whereby both you and the children gradually increase your use of the majority language for all conversations.

PART 4

Language Policies and Politics

18 Language Status, Links to Politics and Racism

We were interested in this topic as, through our discussion with many parents and families over the last six years or so, we have gradually become aware that factors such as attitudes to languages, a passion for a language, and a deep emotional commitment to a language are all far more important than we would have at first assumed in understanding multilingual children and their languages. Although many people would assume that there should be a quite straightforward relationship between the amount and quality of input that a child receives in a particular language, their ability to learn languages and the resulting level of competence that a child acquires, it turns out that it is more complex than that. It also turns out that the relative status and wider visibility of a language, together perhaps with the degree to which adults demonstrate that they care about that language, are also pretty important.

18 Language Status, Links to Politics and Racism

One third of our interviewees were conscious that one language that they spoke was higher status than the other(s). In some cases, a language was perceived as particularly high status (e.g. English in Nigeria), in others, languages had a history of marginalisation (e.g. Welsh, Basque or Kurdish) and/or were linked to racism within a community (which was also likely to affect migrants into Europe). Finally, some differences in status were linked to national language policies.

Languages Perceived as Having High Status

The examples in our sample of languages being perceived as particularly valuable all concerned English. So Adeyinka, who grew up in Nigeria speaking Yoruba at home but English at school commented that, *'People now started to imitate these English, English, English things . . . . You had to be sophisticated and listen to English programmes and English music. . . . We were never encouraged to study Yoruba. People thought if you want to study a language, study English. All the books in Nigeria are in English now. All the preachers, preach in English now. If you speak English it is a very good thing, people respect you if you speak English . . . and if you speak it well. That is what drove people to learn'.*

Similarly, Zwelibanzi, who spoke a mixture of Zulu and English at home, but who spoke exclusively in English at his boarding school, said: *'It was prestigious to talk in English. If you speak English it means you've got guaranteed work because it is an official language'.*

Finally, Rose in Singapore said: *'They speak English in public and they speak as loud as they can, because that means if you speak English you are rich and educated, so therefore it's almost like a social status. Mandarin – you just tick it because you have to tick it, because it's your mother tongue . . . no interest in furthering your mother tongue'.*

Other interviewees described English as being important for doing well in life. This is to be expected for those families living in countries where English is the majority language, but was also the case for those growing up elsewhere, so Bindi's parents sent her to an English-medium primary school in Kenya as they hoped that she would go on to attend university in the UK.

Languages Perceived as Having Lower Status

There were two groups of interviewees who felt that one of their languages was perceived as having low status, the children of those who had migrated from other parts of the world into Europe and those who spoke languages that have been historically or are currently marginalised.

Those who had migrated within Western Europe (i.e. English families living in France, German families living the UK, Spanish families living in Italy or France) did not report any perceived difference in the status of their languages nor did these families encounter overt racism. Those children of migrants who reported experiencing racism were, with one exception, visible minorities (i.e. they looked physically different from the majority population). In most cases, this racism was focused on the children's physical appearance and/or their ethnic origin – it was not directly focused on the language per se. However, this did not stop some children linking their languages and the racism that they experienced.

In Mumtaz's secondary school years, there was racism and bullying. *'We were called Pakis. We wouldn't dare speak our own language . . .as soon as they would hear the words, there would be trouble'.* On the way to and from school, she and her siblings and cousins would go out of their way to avoid a group of adult skinheads who used to hang around in a particular place: *'It was dangerous . . . we were looking over our shoulders'* (see also Vera W's account of racism at school on p.91 and the community reaction to Saadia's family speaking Punjabi and Urdu, p.94).

Mohammed's family from Bangladesh experienced some quite extreme racism while living in London, but the children did not link this to their language or culture. The family were forced to move three times due to racism. They were the only Bengali family on one estate and they were spat on, had dog excrement put through their letterbox, and were told to 'go home'. They finally moved to a house in an area with more Bengali families. Despite this experience of racism, the children valued their culture and continued to speak Bengali/Sylheti. Mohammed says: *'There was no question of the racism we suffered affecting the way we valued our culture'.* They understood that most people were not racist and that it was a small minority who did these things. When Mohammed started secondary school (in 1986), he was allocated to a remedial class in 'Special English' for children who spoke English as a second language. As soon as he started to read – in perfect and fluent English – the teacher sent him back to the main class. It was very clear to Mohammed – who was then aged 11 – that this allocation was done purely on the basis of his ethnicity.

Finally, Tom was the child of migrants who were not part of a visible minority but who still experienced this issue. Tom had moved from Croatia to Australia aged 11, and he remembers being called a 'new Australian', primarily by the Anglo-Saxon group: *'They were giving a hard time to anybody that was not from that background. They called me a "wog" and I remember having an argument. . .I understood it was derogatory. I remember having a fight once because of that. I didn't speak much English, it was fairly early. I was so angry and when the nun came to break up the fight, I remember saying something in Croatian about getting him and killing him and my Croatian friend was translating it into English in the playground. I remember the burst of laughter from other kids. If I had spoken more English I would have probably said that in English to make sure they got the point'.*

The interviewees who said that they experienced racism still reported very positive feelings about their minority culture and language. Although Tom used Croatian less and less in his twenties and thirties, after a gap he returned to the language in later life and is now raising his son bilingually in English and Croatian. Saadia's experience never affected her desire to speak Punjabi or Urdu and she has chosen to speak to her husband in Urdu, and is raising her child speaking Urdu with input in English only from school and the community. Vera W and Mumtaz did decide not to raise their children bilingually. None of these interviewees were those who said that they felt that they did not belong anywhere or were not sure where they belonged.

Interviewees Speaking Marginalised or Oppressed Languages

There were six interviewees growing up speaking languages that were or are marginalised, or were perceived as having low status. These were Basque in Spain, Welsh in the UK, Kurdish in Iraq, Frisian in Holland, Spanish in Texas, and Occitan in France.

Josune spoke Basque at home and at school and Spanish in the community and from watching TV, and felt that she was a balanced bilingual by the age of 10. She attended one of the first schools that offered education in Basque and said that her generation was the first to learn to write in the language. Her mother had a very strict Basque only at home policy. However, as a teenager Josune started to speak more Spanish: 'Everything related to school was in Basque, greetings were in Basque, all topics regarding boys were in Spanish. Basque was undervalued, the Basque people were always regarded as peasants in the community, and it felt more trendy to speak Spanish'. Later in the interview, though, Josune also said that Basque was a language that needed support, but because she had reacted badly to her mother's insistence that she speak Basque at home, she said that she only realised later in adulthood that: '... you needed to look after it, but a teenager does not see it that way. In a way we do have a responsibility of keeping our language, but at the end of it there is a limit, how far you take it within the family....to make it an issue, to create a conflict...' Josune feels that Basque is more valued today than it was when she was growing up: 'I can see there is more confidence in younger people to speak Basque among themselves'. There are TV programmes in Basque, which she thinks makes a huge difference, especially to teenagers who look up to their role models: 'If you see trendy characters speaking in Basque, that's what you do'.

Marion's experience was more like that of a migrant as she was growing up in London speaking a mixture of Welsh and English, where she said: 'Being in London and being Welsh you were mocked. There was a rhyme: "Taffy was a Welshman, taffy was a thief, taffy came to our house and stole a leg of beef. I went to taffy's house, taffy was in bed, I took him by his left leg"....something like that. They sing that to you in the playground, there was a lot of prejudice, there is still prejudice, but it was much more open. No teacher stopped it. It was normal'.

As recounted earlier (see p.111), the negative attitude to Welsh people and Marion's bilingual Welsh background and ways of speaking seem to have had a significant and damaging impact on her educational progress. Marion's family moved to Cardiff when she was 11 where, for the first time, she was not teased and where she felt 'normal'. Within a year all her educational problems were resolved and she went on to become a professor of English literature.

Saad grew up speaking Kurdish at home, and Arabic at school and in the community in Baghdad in Iraq. At the time, Kurdish rebels were fighting against the Iraqi government. The situation was very tense and many Iraqi Arabs were very nationalist and very hostile to the Kurds. Although there was a clear link between the Kurdish language and the Kurdish ethnic group, the Kurdish language was never banned in Iraq (unlike Turkey). Despite this difficult environment, the family did not try to hide their Kurdish identity and Saad would never deny his origin (and as a young adult refused to join the Arab nationalist party, which was a high-risk thing to do at the time). Saad was at school with his two older sisters. One, who was seven years older than Saad, was quite a gentle person, and when people bullied her he would go and defend her. Some teachers were also Arabic nationalists and anti-Kurdish. Saad would be beaten, even when he had not done anything wrong, because of being Kurdish. This negative environment did not affect Saad's willingness or ability to speak Kurdish.

Helen grew up speaking English and Dutch in Holland, but also learnt some Frisian from her grandmother. Helen remembers being embarrassed speaking Frisian as she felt that she was not expected to speak it – she is also aware that Frisian is generally looked down on in Holland and is seen as a rural and somewhat backward language. Although Helen can still understand some Frisian, she cannot speak it today, which she regrets.

Pedro grew up in mostly bilingual and segregated Spanish/English speaking Texas. The community was essentially split in two, with English speakers living in one district with their own church and cinema, and Spanish speakers living in other districts, also with their own church and cinema. A few of the richer white families did not speak Spanish, and despite the huge amount of Spanish spoken locally, surprisingly these white children did not learn very much Spanish at all. Pedro explains that Spanish was a low-status language and that there was a high degree of social separation. There was also outright racism against Spanish speakers. Good jobs would go to white Texans regardless of ability. White Texans would refer to Spanish speakers and those with Spanish surnames inaccurately and insultingly as 'Mexicans'. This bilingual community did not extend to official settings which all operated in English, including the education system, where students who spoke Spanish were punished. There were two parallel schools, with the children of Spanish-speaking families sent to a different and less well resourced but still English-language primary school. All children raised in Spanish-speaking families were held back one year regardless of how well they spoke English. Despite the fact that Pedro could read before starting school, he was still held back one year and enrolled for an introductory preschool year. Later on in school, the children were 'streamed' according to their language background or ethnicity, with white English-speaking children in the top streams (even those who failed years at school), rich children from Hispanic families in the next stream, and poorer Hispanic children in the lower streams. Pedro describes the teachers as having a very negative attitude to Spanish.

It is interesting that, in this negative environment, Pedro and his brother reacted in opposite ways – whilst his brother conformed, Pedro rebelled: *'Anywhere in the school ground you could not speak Spanish. . . .They'd give you a detention. I got a paddling [beating] many times for speaking Spanish. . . . I was always a rebel. I spoke Spanish. You can't tell me not to speak Spanish'.* In fact, there were occasions when Pedro and his friends were speaking English together and when they saw a teacher coming they would switch into Spanish, just to make a point.

Despite this heavily negative attitude, Pedro continued to speak Spanish: *'Nowadays they do bilingual education from a young age, but when I was a kid they actually prevented you from speaking Spanish, which made you speak it even more!'* Pedro's elder brother never rebelled, but instead conformed and spoke English. Despite the brothers' different reactions, Pedro does not feel that this had any impact on the level of his and his brother's Spanish, which is the same.

The last of these interviewees who speak marginalised languages is Sophie, who grew up in south-west France speaking French, Spanish and Occitan. Occitan has some similarities in vocabulary and grammar to Spanish, Italian and Portuguese. Linguists regard it as a distinct language, but in France it is commonly seen either as a dialect or a degraded version of French. This view of the language and the associated cultural and political context had a big impact on Sophie and the languages that she speaks today. *'Occitan is a language which has been, kind of, pushed away . . . it's not considered a language. If you think of Welsh about 50 years ago that is how it is. My father and grandfather had both been forbidden from speaking it . . . My father told us stories about being beaten up at school by teachers because he spoke Occitan with his friends. They would speak it amongst themselves but if they were overheard they were beaten. He was the last generation that spoke it. . . My parents' generation would still speak Occitan in public [e.g. at the market] – with people of their generation, not younger people. If they were speaking Occitan in public and a tourist or a stranger came along they would switch to French'.*

Sophie feels that her situation was quite unusual: *'I don't think in my generation that there were many people who were exposed to [Occitan] as much as I was. My friends at school did not understand it as I did. I think this was because I grew up living with my grandparents which most of my friends did not. Also I had a great uncle who had written poetry and books in Occitan which had been published. . . . I know that but it is not a subject which is very much talked about in my family so I don't know all the details'.*

She also remembers that there were some political issues linked to the language, and that her parents did not want to get involved in this. *'My parents didn't want to get involved with them [cultural events in Occitan]. They never explicitly said why . . . but it's not difficult to work out. . . . I remember going with them when I was about seven to a little concert, music and singing in Occitan. And I remember my father saying at the end of it that he didn't want us to come back to these events, because it was too political'.*

Sophie feels that there was *'anger within the community, a push to create something which didn't work'*. She doesn't believe that there was ever any violence, but she mentions that people were aware of the Basque uprising. Her parents did not want to get involved with any of these initiatives or movements. *'We were growing up in the middle of this. I think that it is only as an adult and living in England where there are policies on ethnic minorities and languages that I began to understand a little bit more about my upbringing and culture, and I think that that is why my sister (who still lives in France) doesn't see it in the same way as me. I started looking into this more recently and through the internet I found out this subject is a very sensitive subject in the community and it is referred to in Occitan as "The big shame". I had never heard this expression as a child or when I was growing up. In France there is just silence . . . it doesn't exist. When I read [this on the internet] I was shocked, but in fact, it does fit in with my experience'.*

Sophie is aware that, even within her own family, the use of Occitan is decreasing: *'When I lived with my family, my parents and their parents would speak in Occitan. I have one grandfather still alive and now, even he does not speak Occitan to his son (my father)'*. Now Sophie is proud of her Occitan heritage but, as a child, she says: *'It wasn't presented as something positive, not because of my family but because of the cultural context . . . the social context'*.

As an adult Sophie speaks French, Spanish, Italian and English fluently. However, she does not feel able to speak Occitan, other than the odd phrase mixed in to a sentence in another language: *'I don't speak Occitan anymore although I understand it. I listen to it occasionally out of nostalgia'*. Sophie does not have an Occitan accent in French, but she does have a French accent when she speaks Occitan. Sophie's sister spoke less Occitan than she did, although she understands it and today they speak Occitan very rarely: *'Occasionally we'll use it but as a joke or a tease. It's a little bit ambivalent and it's a heavily charged language'*.

Of these six interviewees, all except Sophie speak, read and write the marginalised language today. Saad and Josune speak it on a daily basis, whereas for Marion and Pedro it is more occasional. Saad and Josune are both clearly very committed to Kurdish and Basque respectively. Both have opted to raise their children speaking these languages rather than less vulnerable alternatives. Saad is married to an English woman and is raising his children speaking mainly Kurdish and English. Josune is married to a Czech man and lives in England, and is raising her children to speak Basque, Czech and English. Both have decided that the majority and higher status language in the context of their childhoods (Arabic and Spanish) is a lower priority for them. Marion is very committed to her Welsh identity, still uses Welsh regularly, although not daily, and has children but decided not to raise them speaking Welsh. Pedro speaks Spanish now only occasionally, although he is keen to use it more. He did not raise either of his daughters to speak Spanish. Sophie does not have children but says that, if she does, she will raise them multilingually in the other languages she speaks fluently, but not to speak Occitan.

PART 5

Interviewees as Adults

19 Advantages and Disadvantages of Having Been Raised Bilingually

20 One Thing You Would Change about Your Bilingual Childhood and Advice to a Family just Starting Out

21 Low Input and Language Loss and Retention

22 Identities

23 Studying and Working Abroad as Young Adults, Choosing Where to Live More Permanently and Using Bilingualism at Work

24 Relationships

25 Raising Children Monolingually or Bilingually and the Reasons Given

26 Access to Culture as Adults

27 Accents

28 Learning Additional Languages

In this part of the book I explore aspects of our interviewees' lives as adults. This information may seem slightly more removed than that in previous sections from decisions that parents need to make when their children are younger. However, several aspects of the interviewees' reflections on their lives as adults are directly relevant. Many interviewees make links back from what is happening now to their childhoods and, in particular, their view that they are very glad that they were raised bilingually is often informed by the way that their languages and their multilingual world view has proved useful or valuable to them in their adult life. Nonetheless, many of the chapters in this section have more general conclusions (not in bullet form) and, where this is the case, they are probably more of interest in forming a fully-rounded picture of how things turned out, and to provide some additional motivation to keep going when times are tough, rather than having any direct bearing on a specific decision you may need to make as your child(ren) grow(s) up. Some chapters within this section consist of nothing but advice in interviewees' own words to parents, and here again no conclusions are drawn (these include Chapter 19, on advantages and disadvantages, and Chapter 20 on what interviewees would change and their advice to families just setting out).

Interviewees ranged in age from their early twenties to their nineties. Some were married and had started families, some had not. We know from our older interviewees that ways in which languages are used and appreciated continues to change throughout life. It is not a case of children reaching 18 and then being fixed in terms of which languages they use for the rest of their lives. All of our interviewees reached adulthood fluent in two or three languages, and although their use of some these languages may have fallen away, most found that they could still speak them when given the opportunity to do so. Some of the interviewees had retained languages and still spoke them as adults, despite the fact that their input was very limited for large swathes of their childhoods. In other cases, the reduced input had led to the partial or total loss of the language. In this section, I also discuss identities, deciding where to live, bilingualism and work, relationships, accents, learning additional languages and what bilingual adults decided to do in terms of raising their own children.

I start off with what our interviews said, as adults looking back at their childhoods, about the advantages and disadvantages of having been raised bilingually.

19 Advantages and Disadvantages of Having Been Raised Bilingually

Overall, interviewees were overwhelmingly positive about having been raised bilingually. Of our 43 interviewees, 38 made very positive statements about how they were glad to have had the opportunity to grow up using more than one language. No one said that they wished that they had not been raised bilingually. Many would have changed specific aspects of their bilingual upbringing – wished their parents had insisted more (or less), wished that they had kept attending Saturday school, or wished that they had learnt to read and write (see the section on 'One thing you would change about your bilingual childhood'). Only eight interviewees reported any disadvantages at all of having been raised bilingually (and in all cases, specifically pointed out that these were outweighed by the advantages). Three interviewees appeared to us either less positive or more ambivalent about having been raised bilingually (this involved me reading between the lines somewhat, none of them said so explicitly). These were Marion, Mumtaz and Fatima, all of whom faced considerable difficulties as children. In Mumtaz's case, her mother's ill-health was a factor that took a deep toll on the whole family and thus although moving to the UK aged seven and the fact that neither of her parents spoke good English did complicate things, it was not at all the root problem in her life. For Fatima, the move from Morocco aged 10 and the interruption to her education has had an impact on her, but she was already bilingual before she left Morocco and, for her, it was the timing and nature of the move that was the problem, and not speaking three languages. Marion's early problems were more directly linked to the disagreements over languages in her Welsh/English family, but in her case, these were resolved by the time she was 10 years old and she has gone on to have a very successful career. All three of these interviewees clearly deeply value both the languages that they speak, but all three said things that suggested that they had found the process more difficult than the rest of our interviewees.

I will look at what interviewees gave as the advantages of being raised multilingually first.

Advantages

The advantages suggested by interviewees can be roughly divided into three groups: more practical advantages, advantages in terms of relationships and advantages linked to ways of thinking or different world views.

Amongst the practical advantages were the fact that being bilingual had helped with passing exams, getting jobs and advancing careers, and also with learning additional languages (see p.199). For Ingrid (in Sweden speaking English and Swedish), being bilingual helped because everyone in Sweden learns English: *'When we studied my classmates would struggle in English literature. They would spend hours ... looking things up and I felt really fortunate that I didn't have to. When we had English speaking lecturers in Sweden, I would ask questions, and never needed to worry about the language'.*

Many interviewees mentioned that their various languages had been useful for work in terms of higher earnings or greater ease in finding work. Sometimes this was just the ability to speak a useful language, but at a higher level others, such as Sylvia, felt that that being bilingual may have helped her to think abstractly which was important in her degree and her career: *'Being a bilingual you tended to be able to understand concepts beyond what was in language ... There might be concepts that were easy to describe in one language and not the other or that somehow you could reach at ...'* (there are more examples of interviewees using languages in their careers and jobs – see the section on work, p.173).

Similarly, when asked how she feels now about being raised bilingually, Camilla said: *'It's the best thing. It's such a huge part of my identity. Now I work in English [as an editor] and I think that's down to having two languages. I think I understand language in a different way'.* Four of our interviewees also did work that involved manipulating one language in very sophisticated ways; Marion is a professor of English Literature, Camilla edits English written texts and Parvati is a writer, journalist and editor. Tom combined his technical and science background with communication skills and developed a successful career as a technical author / writer. Several years ago he received a prize from the British Institute of Scientific and Technical Communicators for the clarity and effective presentation of information in a technical manual he wrote.

Other interviewees mentioned that knowing two languages was important for keeping up relationships; for Christine, for instance, this meant that she could stay in touch with her relatives in Germany. She is in regular touch with her German relatives, most of whom do not speak French or English and who she speaks to in German. Some interviewees at a fundamental level contrasted how, as children growing up bilingually, they had avoided the problems sometimes associated with learning a language as a foreign language. Saad said, *'[As an adult], I started to study Spanish ... the effort and the hours you put when you are an adult ... and the money. But when you are child and someone just speaks to you ...you don't even realise [you are learning it] ...'.*

The interviewees' comments referring to bilingualism as having given them access to different ways of thinking or more or enhanced world views are quite striking. So, for example, Mohammed said: *'I think that bilingualism is a real blessing, it just gives you a completely different vantage point, a different perspective on the world. And a different perspective of the power of words. . . . I live in that grey area, neither one thing nor another. Bilingual people are simultaneously insiders and outsiders and I think that's a lot more powerful than being one or another'.*

Parvati said: *'I love it. It gives me a sense of another level of understanding, because language orders our sense of ourselves in the world. It dictates our morality and how we can express our feelings and I think that once you have two languages, you can do that in a more sophisticated way because you can access levels of meaning, . . . And because that language contains within it a system of looking at life and death . . .it's really useful. In Hindi the word for yesterday is the same as the word for tomorrow, it's the same word. In English we have the past, present and the future. In Hindi, it's not linear, it's circular, the Hindi cycle of life can be expressed in that one word. . . . Your whole view of the way the world works is formed through language'.*

Claudia said: *'I think that there are huge advantages to being bilingual. . . . I think it's really nice because it opens up a completely different world. . . . There are certain things that I could never explain to an English person in English. Because it's a very German thing, I would need to explain it in German to a German person'.*

Is it a coincidence that there were two therapists in our group of 40 or so interviewees? Or are the two therapists right when they said that bilingualism makes for an enriched person? *'You are more open minded in understanding others'*, and *'I think it has shaped my brain. . . . It made me creative, in trying to work out what people are saying . . . you acquire acute hearing, I think, when you are bilingual'.*

Several other interviewees mentioned that it made them more sensitive to different cultures. Pedro from Texas in the United States said: *'. . .being bilingual helps you accept different cultures and customs . . . you respect them because you've got customs of your own, and a lot of Americans, they just don't get it . . .'.* Kwesi said, *'When you go somewhere you are sensitive to the local culture, you can pick up things more easily, because if you know only one language and live only in one place when you go abroad you have only one frame of reference. Having different languages allowed me to go travelling and also to have more frames of reference'.*

Finally in this group, Isabelle said: *'It was great [being raised bilingually]. It was quite complicated because of what happened with my parents. But it is valuable. I think your imaginary world is much richer. You have cultural experiences and cultural references, and so a richer inner life. I've never not had it. . . . It is a gift to be able to understand several languages'.*

Disadvantages

As mentioned above, eight interviewees identified a possible or actual disadvantage of being raised bilingually, although each one also said that the advantages outweighed the disadvantage that they reported. The most common disadvantage identified was that being raised bilingually may have meant that the interviewees did not have a perfect grasp of both languages. Some of them were told this as children and this feeling has lingered on, so, as we quoted in the chapter on education (p.126), at school Ingrid *'was told a couple of times by teachers – "Well you speak two languages OK but not one perfectly"'.* Other interviewees gave specific examples of ways in which they felt that one or more of their languages were deficient. Shadi with her four languages said: *'And I don't think that you can speak any of these languages perfectly. The other day, my children had to do these similes "as cold as . . . ice" and I couldn't do half of them. . . . In French, because I haven't spoken it except with my children for a long time, I can't remember how to say things and I have to look them up in the dictionary. . . . At work when I'm writing reports, sometimes*

I am disadvantaged in my writing, I have to look things up, or someone uses an everyday word that I have not heard before, and I don't understand it'.

As mentioned above (see p.34), Camilla, who speaks Danish and English, is aware that she still makes mistakes in English that she has inherited from her Danish mother, although the examples that she gives are ones that I feel perhaps only a professional editor would notice.

Claudia also felt that: *'I think that the only disadvantage [of being bilingual] is that you can end up not speaking both languages 100%. That's the one disadvantage. . . . My English vocabulary is OK but there are some English words that I don't know. If I compare myself to some monolingual English speakers I know, they will occasionally use a word I don't know'.* Claudia did acknowledge that the people she was comparing herself were unusually adept with language, and that this did not necessarily mean that her English was not on a par with a monolingual of her background, educational level and intelligence. Nonetheless, Claudia mentioned, for example, that she quite often struggles with the low-value questions on the show 'Who Wants to be a Millionaire' which frequently use proverbs, idioms, nursery rhymes and other common everyday cultural knowledge.

The only other possible disadvantage of bilingualism identified by interviewees resulted from the fact that bilingualism is often linked to frequent moves or living away from 'home'. Thus Sylvia said: *'Perhaps I'm also saying it's great to be bilingual especially if you want an international life but an international life can be lonely rather than glamorous. If that's not what you want, bilingualism can be a little over-rated (nice and good for holidays). I wouldn't say that bilingualism is a mixed blessing because it really has no down-sides for me at all but there is a danger of allowing the gift to rule one's life'.*

As mentioned above, some other interviewees mentioned feeling *'rootless'* (e.g. Shadi), or sometimes feeling, like Sabina, that they did not really belong anywhere *'which is quite hard to deal with'* (see also Chapter 22 on Identities, p.165).

20 One Thing You Would Change about Your Bilingual Childhood and Advice to a Family Just Starting Out

We also asked all of our interviewees what advice they would give to a family just starting out and to specify one thing that, if they could go back, they would change about their own bilingual childhood. In many cases these two answers covered similar areas, so both sets of responses are included here. They are useful in bringing together in one section many of the diverse issues that we have raised throughout the book. In some areas there were no contradictions between the answers, although in other areas interviewees did have diverging or even opposing views.

Starting with the more general comments, five interviewees simply said, 'speak your own language to your children'. So Shadi (living in England), said: *'Always speak to your child first and foremost in your mother tongue. With my children until they were two or three, I only spoke to them in Farsi but I read to them in French, and they had videos and DVDs and music in French. Later I started speaking to them in French at the weekends and now I use it more day-to-day'.*

Two interviewees mentioned the need to start early. Charles, for instance, emphasised the need to start very early: *'Start from day one! Even during pregnancy I was speaking to my partner's stomach in French! From the moment of conception'.*

Twelve interviewees referred to the need to *'keep going'* or to *'persevere'*. Vera W said: *'Keep it up. Don't lose your language, your traditions, your culture. Make sure your children know about it. My eldest son was doing an assembly based on Chinese New Year, and suddenly he got quite interested in it. I was quite sad that he was interested in it because school was doing it, rather than because I had taught him'.*

The idea of perseverance implies that you are up against some difficulties, and several interviewees referred to this. Some mentioned the external environment not always being helpful or supportive: *'Keep the multilingualism and speak your language to your child. . . . It will be difficult. Usually, the surrounding environment will not understand. The education environment might not either'.* And Christine said: *'Stick at it, because it's not always easy. It is very easy to give up, especially when they start school . . . homework is in English, TV is in English. If you want your children to be bilingual you have to work at it'.* Others, like Saadia, mentioned that, at times, progress might seem to be very slow: *'No matter how little you think you're doing, no matter how little the improvement is, the best option is just to persevere and the results will show . . . in a big bang down the line. Just keep at it'.*

Some linked the issue of perseverance with consistency. Rose, for whom both the parent and the school language had switched over during her childhood from Mandarin to English because of a change in national language policy in Singapore, said: '... *persist and be consistent ...'* and Armelle said: *'Speak your mother tongue to your children. Never switch. Never ever'*. Of course it may take a certain discipline to be consistent. Bindi, for example, said that: *'When my children attended Gujarati school, parents who came to pick up their children would speak to them in English, why send them to Gujarati school if you are going to speak to them in English, at least try to speak to them in Gujarati ... be conscious about that, be disciplined about it. I speak to my children in Gujarati at their [mainstream English-medium] school. I think that that is important that they understand that, that they feel comfortable, confident in that language'*.

We now come to the difficult area of how much parents should be prepared to push a language with their children. Interviewees were not agreed on this. Many interviewees giving advice to others felt that parents should try to make children's exposure to a second language very natural and part of daily life. However, particularly when looking back on their own childhoods, some wondered if their parents should not have pushed them a little more.

So in the first group, (Hindi and English-speaking) Parvati said: *'Just naturally speak, through a kind of osmosis, rather than forcing children to go to school when their friends are playing football. Not everyone might agree with this but, for me, this meant that I came back to it as an adult – hence my decision to learn Sanskrit at university'*. Ingrid (who did not reply to her mother in Swedish throughout her childhood) said: *'I am very grateful that my mother persisted in her very mellow way ... Don't pressure your children and just keep the languages alive and just make it part of daily life and not a chore or a struggle'*. You may remember Josune, who felt that her mother's insistence on her children speaking exclusively Basque at home was a source of conflict within the family. In her case, and as a result of her own experience, she would never tell children off for using one language over the other. She feels very strongly about this and thinks that parents should not impose it on their children. If children are pushed into speaking the mother tongue it will cause resentment. Although Bindi has deliberately gone to some lengths to ensure that her children speak both Gujarati and English, she is also cautious about this area: *'As [my children] get older, it is getting more and more difficult and they are speaking more English. We have decided to stop constantly reminding them, as it feels like nagging [and may be counter productive] and we are hoping that they will come back to it on their own when they are a bit older ...'*.

In contrast, in the second group, Camilla who did not reply to her parents in Danish after she had started school, said: *'I **wish** my parents had persevered a bit more and said to me "When you are at home speak Danish to us" but I don't know, I might have been unhappy ... I might have really rejected it. It's such a huge part of who I am. I have such a soft spot for Denmark, I really idealise it. I think you have to go individually with what your child wants. I don't think that you should push it too hard, but I do think that they could have **tried** to push it a little bit. Personally I don't think it's worth pushing it if it makes your child unhappy, if they're unhappy at school or if they feel like a stranger or if there is a risk that they will reject it.*

But there are such huge benefits that it's worth trying to keep it as much as you can'. With her own child Sabina has developed her own form of 'gentle pushing': *'What I do is if my son says a sentence to me in Urdu but inserts one word in English, I ask him the word in Urdu and usually he knows it. And I think that that works – a little bit of pushing … a gentle form of pushing'.* Of her own childhood, Sabina also wonders if: *'Maybe [it would have been good] if I had been pushed into reading and writing a bit. I don't know how I would have reacted and whether I would have accepted it, though'.*

However, another group of four interviewees felt that the whole issue of whether or how much to push children could be avoided if exposure to a second language was a fun experience, and they said that parents should avoid making it a chore. Although this seems to make a lot of sense, this is not something that comes across from the interviewees' own childhoods, and it may be more difficult to put into practice than it sounds. Mohammed said: *'Make sure kids have access to books in both languages. Make sure the books are not burdensome, they should be fun. You need to create a love of language in children … endless stories. Then they will learn later. It's not about academic or formal learning'.* Josune also explained how she went to some trouble to ensure that her children associate Basque (their third language) with having fun: *'In my case my children relate Basque to their cousins, summer with a swimming pool, lots of friends and freedom to play outdoors, and my relatively large lively family. They have a lot of fun out there. I make sure that they spend time there on their own without us (they would speak English to us otherwise) so that they can be sucked into the culture. This has enabled them to develop a positive and enthusiastic attitude towards Basque, despite me not speaking to them that much nowadays due to time pressures, and them not having anyone else in the UK with whom they can speak Basque'.*

After all, as Adeyinka said: *'I would try to raise children so that they have a fascination for that culture. Because you can teach them and speak it to them … but they have to **want** to speak it'.*

Another group of eight interviewees talked about the importance of learning to read and write in both languages. Mohammed said of his own childhood: *'I would have hoped that I could have kept up my Bengali and Arabic in a way that would have meant that I could read in Bengali and Arabic for pleasure. I wish I had an appreciation of those languages – from novels to music to art – I didn't get access to the whole culture – it was more about formal learning and gave me a top-heavy view of the language. I think that my parents could have done more to cultivate a love of those languages, rather than feeling that learning the language was a necessity'.* And Saadia said: *'I would change the fact that I didn't keep going to Saturday school. I wish that I had learnt much more and I wish that I was much more confident in Urdu especially reading and writing. I wish I had also learnt to read Punjabi. I could have done GCSE Urdu …'.* More specifically, one interviewee mentioned that it is important that children start Saturday school when they are relatively young.

Four interviewees said that they would change absolutely nothing about their bilingual childhoods.

Adeyinka (Yoruba and English) wished that both his parents had spoken the same dialect of their local language so that he could have learnt that and become trilingual. Pedro (speaking Spanish in Texas) and Sophie (speaking Occitan in France) both wished that there had been less linguistic discrimination. Snjezana wished that she had realised as a child that the discrimination within her bilingual school was their problem (and not hers). Isabelle wished that more dual or bilingual societies existed like Quebec in Canada, where being bilingual is the norm and not the exception. Christine and Charles both wished that their mothers had not stopped speaking French and Dutch to them respectively. Two interviewees living in the UK wished that their own parents had been able to learn more English. One interviewee wished that her move to the UK from abroad had taken place when she was younger, so that she could have done better in the education system. Marion, who felt her family was divided by language, advised parents to avoid this at all costs. Parvati would have liked both of her parents to be equally supportive of both languages (which they both spoke): *'I would like them to have decided the level that we were going to be exposed to that language [Hindi]. ... My father has this snobbery, which I think we initially inherited, but soon discarded about speaking Hindi being a bit low class, I would liked to have changed that. My father left it to my mother and always sneered at it a bit'.*

One interviewee's advice was a useful reminder that all children are different, and that parents should not expect each child in a family to react in the same way. One interviewee strongly recommended that parents try to send their children to school in the second language because *'there is only so much you can do from home'.* Other advice included reminding children of how important it is for them to be able to communicate with their monolingual relatives, and going to visit such relatives or a country speaking their minority language every year or regularly.

Finally, Sophie, who is now a clinical psychologist, said: *'My observations of children, and having worked with bilingual children, and with my experience of having this taken away from me, has taught me that it's crucial to pass it on – because you have to make children aware what they are and what they come from. I have met so many adults where one of the adults is from one culture and they didn't speak that language .... I think it is ridiculous to think that you are hurting a child by talking a foreign language to them. It's by making it a shameful thing that you are hurting them. I think that it's important for the two parents to be positive about the languages'.*

21 Low Input and Language Loss and Retention

It was quite surprising to us how many of our sample had kept on speaking languages despite input that dropped to very low levels for sustained periods, whereas my assumption would have been that, in all of these cases, the languages in question would have been very quickly lost. In some cases, languages <u>were</u> lost and parents should certainly not aim to follow these examples. I have pulled together some information on these examples here. I hope that this will give parents going through difficult times some hope. This section also highlights how different children are, and how important emotional factors are in terms of motivating children to continue to use languages or not.

Languages Retained Despite Low Input

Five interviewees retained languages that they stopped having much significant exposure to. Christine was initially raised speaking German and French in France. Christine's mother stopped speaking German to her (apart from the odd word) when she was around six. After this, Christine's exposure to German was limited to family holidays to visit monolingual German-speaking relatives in Germany. These holidays took place at least once a year and sometimes more, and they occasionally lasted several weeks. Christine had no other input from books, TV, films or videos, or any other German-speaking friends or contacts. Christine did attend beginners' German lessons at school (although she did not find these very inspiring). Despite this, Christine has retained her German – she still visits her relatives in Germany and uses it then. As an adult, she worked in both Germany and Switzerland and also used German professionally in the UK. Christine does not read German books or watch German films and she regrets this. She has some German friends that she has met in the UK, but she tends to speak English to them.

Astrid is an even more extreme example because her (German) parents spoke to her in English in Australia, but she learnt German through a six-month stay in Germany when she was around four years old. After that she attended an all-day German Saturday school for three years, starting when she was seven until she was around 10 years old. She then stopped speaking or hearing German at all apart from beginners' secondary school classes and a language degree at university. Despite this, she still speaks German and is raising her son to speak German. Her parents have now moved back from Australia to Germany and she now speaks to them in German as well.

Fatima moved from Morocco to the UK when she was 10. In Morocco she spoke Arabic at home, but her school was bilingual in French and Arabic. After arriving in the UK, Fatima had no continuing input in French apart from the secondary school beginners' French classes but she retained her French and is still comfortable speaking it today, although she says that she has few opportunities to do so.

Daniela spoke Italian and English with her parents, but she was sent to a boarding school in Switzerland when she was eight where she learnt French, which was the only language any of the children were allowed to speak at any time. She stayed at the school for only three years until she returned to the UK when she was 11 and went to an English boarding school. Here she had beginners' French lessons with the other children, which she did not enjoy, and her mother hired French au pairs to help her to keep up her French. These were the only forms of input in French that Daniela had after the age of 11, but she is still quite confident in using French to do a range of tasks from speaking and listening to writing letters.

Finally, Isabelle retained her English after moving aged nine after her parents' divorce from Atlanta to France where she only spoke English to her brother who was several years younger than she was. As she had a considerable emotional attachment to English, she also continued to read in English, listened to English radio and wrote to her father in English. Nonetheless the content of the English that she spoke must have been quite limited. She never felt that she lost her fluency in English although she had to work hard to be able to use written English at school after she returned to the United States to live with her father aged 17.

Language Partially Lost But Then Reactivated

Some interviewees had some early input in a language before losing their fluency in speaking it, but they were still able to reactivate it later through study or travel. This includes Isabelle, who had heard Polish from her grandparents until the age of six when her family moved away and she saw her grandparents much less frequently. She had no further input in Polish. Nonetheless, she opted to study it at university and after several language courses was able to join a programme studying Polish culture, and she was able to go to Poland to study. Isabelle still uses her Polish today, and is quite confident in most tasks.

Charles's story was quite similar to Christine's in that his mother had spoken some Dutch and some French to him, but stopped speaking Dutch to him as a child. Until he was eight he also attended a school that used Dutch, German and French as language media. However, after this, Charles's input in Dutch was very limited (to the odd word at home and 'boring' language classes at school). When Charles decided to go to Holland to do his Masters and PhD (which he would be studying and writing in English), his Dutch was basic. When he started living in Holland his Dutch became much better, and by the time he left his Dutch had improved considerably, and he felt more comfortable speaking it. Now, although Charles considers English and French his dominant languages, he is still very confident speaking and reading Dutch, although he is less confident writing in it.

Finally in this section, Daniela features again – this time regarding her Italian. Daniela had started speaking Italian as a very young child living in Italy with an English mother and an Italian father. When her parents divorced and her mother moved back to the UK when Daniela was four, the English nanny her mother hired could not understand Daniela as she spoke mostly or totally in Italian. Although Daniela's mother spoke some Italian, she did not continue to speak any to Daniela after they returned to the UK, and so after the age of four Daniela's input in Italian was limited to periodic visits to her father and his family in Italy. For a period of four years from when she was between the ages 10 and 14 she did not see her father at all, and their only contact was occasional phone calls (when Daniela spoke in English). During this period, her father moved to France and when Daniela did visit him there after she was 14, they spoke in French. Daniela feels: *'I can understand Italian really well, and my Italian is OK, I can speak reasonably OK, it's still almost at that childish level, because that was the kind of Italian that I learnt, so when I go back to Italy, each time it's developing and becoming more mature in the way that I speak'.* Several months prior to talking to our interviewer, Daniela went to Rome with her eight-year-old daughter and her English husband to visit her Italian cousins for the first time after ten years. *'They were surprised that I could still remember some Italian, and that I could still speak in Italian and my husband, he's never really heard me speak Italian...I was quite fluent to him, because he has no concept of it, and he was going "Your Italian is great!", he was really impressed by my Italian, certainly didn't think that I spoke with a very English accent!'*

Daniela is sure that the visit to Italy was a 'catalyst'. She felt really good when she spoke Italian in Italy again after 10 years: *'Getting back to my roots and thinking: "Oh I really miss that Italian side of me!"'* She also surprised herself that she could still speak Italian fluently if needed after a gap as long as ten years: *'We were in a taxi on the way to the hotel and the cab driver was driving like a maniac and he was also on a mobile phone, driving really fast and we had our daughter in the back of the car....I just suddenly turned to him and said in Italian: "I think that's enough! That is very dangerous, I have a child in the back seat!" And he was so shocked, he put his phone down straight away! I was angry; it just came out, without thinking! And I thought "Oh, that was interesting, where did that come from?!" So it is there...it is in my head...'.*

Languages (Partially) Lost

Two interviewees did seem to have left languages along the way, at least in terms of being able to actively speak them rather than passively understand. (In all our cases these were third languages, and so the interviewees had still been raised bilingually.)

Aimee had been raised trilingually in Togo with Kabye at home, Mina predominantly in the community and French at school, until she was eight and moved to France. In France her aunt continued to speak to her in Kabye and she spoke French at school and in the community, but she stopped speaking or hearing Mina at all. She began to lose her Mina, and during holidays to the Ivory Coast, if she spent time in the south (where Mina is the majority language), she would try to speak Mina, but, by this time, she was increasingly comfortable in French and would prefer to speak in French rather than Mina (and eventually also Kabye): *'When I was living in France I could always speak Kabye because we spoke Kabye at home but I did start to lose my Mina'*. Today Aimee does not speak or understand Mina at all.

Sophie was raised speaking French, Occitan and some Spanish in south-western France. In her case, she continued to have input in Occitan from her parents and grandparents at home throughout her childhood – at least until she left home to attend a school that had wider options when she was 15 years old. Sophie retained her French and Spanish (although she had less input in Spanish as a child) and added Italian and English to her languages. However, although she can understand it, she cannot speak Occitan today: *'I don't speak Occitan anymore although I understand it. I listen to it occasionally out of nostalgia'*. In Sophie's case, as Occitan is a language which is now spoken very little – and which UNESCO recognises as endangered – it would be quite hard for her to find other speakers to speak Occitan with. Apart from the fact that she was the only interviewee who had spoken a language which was close to disappearing, one other thing does seem to distinguish Sophie and her family from the other families speaking marginalised and oppressed languages and that is that, because of the particular circumstances in France, her family seem to have internalised society's negative view of the language to a greater extent, or at least seem not to have reacted to it. In the other families, society's negative views seem to have often made the families more proud to be Kurdish, Welsh or Basque and in Pedro's case, more rebellious and more likely to speak Spanish at school, even if that meant getting beaten (again).

Conclusion

All experts would advise that children are given consistent and regular input in all the languages that they are raised speaking, but these examples show that some interviewees were able to retain their languages despite very low levels of input for many years. Interviewees were able to reactivate a language that they had not spoken for many years by visiting or going to live in a country where that language is spoken. Some interviewees did lose languages though, so please do not allow this to make you complacent.

- This tells us that if you have an unavoidable gap in language input for a period of time, this does not mean that all is lost and you can reinvigorate a language again by arranging for input to restart after a gap of months or even years.
- If you do have a gap in input for a period, it is worth trying to arrange even one hour's input a week or a series of visits to where the language is spoken as a majority language (or both). This may not be enough to continue to develop the language, but it may be just enough to retain most of what the child already has.
- Where a child has a strong emotional commitment to a language (e.g. as Isabelle did), conversations with a sibling and/or listening to the radio or TV in that language may well also help a child to retain it.

22 Identities

As there is evidence in the literature that some bilinguals struggle more with issues of identity than monolinguals do, we also asked people about their identity – whether there was a place or a community that they felt that they belonged to, and even what national sports team they supported. This whole area is very complex indeed. Very few (in fact only seven) of the interviewees came down simply on one side of their bilingual identity or the other. More than half told us that they somehow belonged or wanted to belong to both communities or to no community at all. For some this was very positive, while, for others, it felt like something that they struggled with or which made them uncomfortable. Some interviewees had travelled as young adults – seemingly to test out whether they would feel they belonged better in another country where their other language was widely spoken.

Interviewees who had learnt a language purely through attending school were much more likely to have a simple and singular identity – which was always based around the home language rather than that used in school. So, for example, Emilio, who learnt English only through his schooling, says that he is an Argentinean who speaks English. Although he also says that he has a special relationship or link with England, he met his (French) wife in the UK and has spent a considerable portion of his adult life working in London. He even adds that he does not think of himself as bilingual, because he learnt English solely through his bilingual school. Zwelibanzi, who learnt English primarily at school (as well as some from his father), says he has a strong Zulu identity: *'When I introduce myself I always find that I have to say "I'm Zulu"'*. He also says: *'You can learn a language to acquire a skill, or for social life, but when it comes to your identity, when you talk about yourself, you find that you have to speak in your mother tongue. It's a natural thing. Somebody told me "when you cry, it doesn't matter where you are, the first yell you do, you yell in your mother tongue"'*.

Two of the interviewees who had successfully learnt very marginalised languages as children also felt that they belong to those communities, so, for instance, Marion said: *'For me it was a success going back to Wales and I see myself as Welsh not English'*. She feels that Welsh is her emotional language and that she has Welsh values. In sport, Marion supports Wales. Josune's situation is more complex as she has English, Spanish and Basque to contend with, but Josune has been living in England for more than 15 years. She feels closer to England than to Spain, and closer to the English flag than to the Spanish flag. She does not support Spanish sports teams and would be happy if the Basque nation had a team, like Wales and Scotland do: *'Then I would support the Basque team. Many Basque people feel the same'*.

Only three other interviewees clearly identified with one side or the other: Claudia, who grew up moving around the world speaking German and English with her parents who were both German, said that despite the fact that English was now her stronger language (and that she had decided to live in England), her identity is still more German than English. She says that she feels German. Sylvia, who grew up in France as the daughter of English parents, said: *'I am an English person who happened to grow up in France ... I am an English person who has never watched Blue Peter'*. However, elsewhere in the interview, Sylvia was also the interviewee who described feeling like an *'outsider and not belonging anywhere'*, and referred to *'... the misfit syndrome that often comes hand in hand with bilingualism because both come from being a migrant ...'*. She now lives in the UK.

Finally, Armelle, after having a minor 'crisis' about where she belonged after completing university (as described below), has clearly reflected on this and says: *'I feel more "me" in French ... Since we have been in London, and we have seen a lot of my French friends, my husband has told me "when you are with your French friends you act differently" ... My brother tells me that he likes me more in French than in Spanish. I feel more comfortable in French. My [Spanish-speaking] mother knows that and she agrees, and it is not a problem for her'*. Armelle also says: *'When I am angry or I want to swear, I do it in French. If I am upset with someone, but I don't say anything, I think about it in French'*. Despite the fact that she feels more comfortable in French but is married to a Spanish speaker who does not speak very much French (yet), she does not see this as a problem for her relationship at all. She has, after all, decided to live in her husband's Spanish-speaking home country, Argentina, and not in France.

Another group of interviewees described how their identities had shifted over time. So Vera W, who grew up in a Chinese family in the UK, simply says: *'I started off as a small child being very Chinese, but I've kind of lost that now, which is quite sad really. Now I feel more English than Chinese'*. Similarly, Matilde, who went from Italy to Zaire where her parents were working, said: *'Now I feel Italian – by the time I completed my university studies I felt Italian. But when I first came back to Italy from Goma, despite the fact that I had wanted to come back to Italy, I felt that I belonged in Goma, I was fifteen, most of my memories until then had been in Africa and I didn't feel like I belonged in Italy'*.

Camilla can also pinpoint the moment when her identity started to change: *'I felt completely Danish growing up [in England] ... **completely Danish.** And it wasn't until I moved to Denmark for a bit when I was 18, and then I thought "I'm not Danish" and people said to me "You're really English"'*. Now she says: *'It's like I belong somewhere in the middle. I wanted to belong somewhere. And I think that I took the English side. ... Recently I gave up my Danish passport ... and once you've given it up, they won't give it back ... it was quite emotional really'*. But she also says: *'Whenever I've had emotional or personal problems, I always go to Denmark. It's like my sanctuary'*.

Another group of interviewees say that they feel that they belong to all the communities that they have grown up in, so Aimee feels that she is a mixture of influences, including Kabye, French, and English, and she feels comfortable with this. Sarah avoids the question neatly when she says that she feels: *'European. I wouldn't be able to decide whether I was more German or English'*. When asked which language he identifies most closely with, Mohammed said: *'I think in English, but I can articulate those thoughts in Bengali. I form the words in English and I translate them to speak in Bengali. . . . So I am more English. . . . Bangladesh is not my country, it is my history now'*. But, as mentioned above, elsewhere in the interview, he also said: *'I live in that grey area, neither one thing nor another. Bilingual people are simultaneously insiders and outsiders and I think that's a lot more powerful than being one or another'*.

Kwesi, who grew up in Ghana, but in an area where international staff lived where he attended a private school, says: *'Obviously I am Ghanaian and before I came to live and work in England it never occurred to me to be anything else but Ghanaian. But if you live somewhere as part of a minority and people have a certain perception of how you should be, and you don't fit that mould, it makes you think . . . If people say you don't sound like a Ghanaian, you don't act like a Ghanaian, so you think "Hmm, so what do I have to do to become more Ghanaian?" you know, and all these questions come. . . . I used to describe myself as being British West African, this is best to describe a combination of influences of one's upbringing, you know; I often said that my mental constitution, if expressed physically, would be mixed race, because then people wouldn't expect you to be wholly one thing'*. Furthermore, he explains that sometimes he lets people believe their assumptions that he was raised in the UK. It seems easier that way without having to explain his upbringing. Later in the interview he adds words to the effect that he does not see that difference in his identity as negative, as he sees himself as a global citizen; not fitting every box *'. . . which is positive all the way. Everybody should have the opportunity to be exposed to different cultures, act more globally, think more globally'*.

Vera C, our 90-year-old interviewee, simply said: *'When I speak French [as opposed to English], I'm a different being'*, and explains that she feels that she has two separate and different identities, one for each language.

Most of the remaining interviewees either felt that they belonged nowhere or said that they did not believe in the idea of nationality or any one identity. So one interviewee said: *'I just think that it doesn't matter. Anyway this idea of states or countries . . . whatever. . . . I do belong to my set . . . the cards that I have been handed . . .The world doesn't allow for a multiple identity – you need to be one thing or another. The thing about America, most people come from somewhere else, so in that sense I am American. Because my father and brother are there, and because I go back there, I guess America is probably home. But I think if you looked at things in a vacuum, probably the place that I would be most at home is Quebec City because there, there is just no question, you speak French, you speak English and that's normal'*.

Parvati says several different things about this – the first of which is that she does not feel more at home in either India or Britain, and, as a woman, struggles with aspects of life in both countries, but she also says: *'Parts of you that have always been at odds with the mainstream culture, do feel explained when you go to India'*. At another point in the interview she also said: *'I have a strong sense of my Indian identity. But I'm selective about it. I'm not nationalistic about it and I'm not "mother India" about it, if you know what I mean . . .'*.

Snjezana's situation is complicated by changes in the state where she was born: *'What I grew up belonging to (Yugoslavia) no longer exists. My parents always describe themselves as Croatian. When I am asked where I come from, I say Hungary [which is where she was living when the interview took place]. But then they see my surname and then I have to explain. I think definitely my identity has been shaped by my languages; Croatian, Esperanto, and Italian'.* Elsewhere in the interview, when discussing bringing up her son bilingually, Snjezana also comments: *'You can try to assimilate, change your name. But you can't assimilate if the majority community doesn't accept you . . . . My sister always said "My children are Italian in Italy and Croatian in Croatia" but I don't think that works, I tell my child the opposite so "we are Croatian in Hungary and Hungarian in Croatia". I can see why assimilating would be tempting . . .but in my view, better to be different and be proud to be different'.*

Making the point that for many children being bilingual was intimately connected with moving between countries, Swedish and English-speaking Ingrid says: *'I don't really feel rooted anywhere. There is nowhere that is really home. That's the big negative part. But then maybe that's also because we've moved a lot . . .'.*

In Pedro's case, although he did not move as a child, he says that he does not feel at home in his part of Texas because of the social hierarchy, social segregation and racism against Spanish speakers: *'That's why I don't go home. . . . I get too radical when I go home. That's why I left. I couldn't take it. I would probably have been in jail if I had stayed. Some people accept it, but I never did. I was a militant. And it still goes on . . . a lot of whites think that they can do whatever they want . . .'.*

When asked about her identity, Mumtaz says: *'If I go to Pakistan, to them you're English, but when you're here . . . . I personally call myself a British Asian, whereas the older cousins call themselves Pakistani. When you experience racism here, you feel you should be there, but when you are there, you are just a visitor. Personally I feel I belong here. There is no family there now'.* Similarly, Daniela has a mixed view: *'I feel much more at home in Italy, although my Italian family consider me to be very English! In a way, I almost do not belong anywhere, but I feel more at home in Italy than here'.*

Sophie with her Occitan, French and Spanish background said: *'I don't know . . . that's the answer, I don't know. I wouldn't describe myself as Occitan, but it's very important to me to say that I am from the south of France (which is really another way of saying more or less the same thing). It's the ambivalence again because officially [Occitan] doesn't exist; ethnic groups don't exist in France. I have a French passport but I don't feel French either. French in the language I grew up with . . . OK I am French but I am also a lot of other things'.*

Fatima initially answered with one view, but then seemed to wonder if that should imply that she would be happy to live in the country of her choice, which she said she would find difficult to do in the long term: *'I feel more Moroccan. . . . [even though] I speak more English, than Arabic now. Maybe I'm half and half. I would find it hard, I think, to go back and live in Morocco. When I go back I don't always think I belong. It's simple things like queuing. I go to queue and people don't queue – in the UK everyone queues – at the bank, at the shops . . . and people don't do that . . . and that frustrates me. I don't think I could live there – maximum stay is four to five weeks and then it's time to go'.*

Sabina is torn between saying that she belongs to both English and Urdu cultures, or neither. In her case, the fact that she speaks Urdu but is not a practising Muslim is a barrier to belonging to the Urdu-speaking community: *'I think I am a mixture of both. I think in terms of the language and fluency, English is far more dominant, my thinking is in*

English ... Sometimes I feel that I don't really belong anywhere which is quite hard to deal with ... I think I've got pockets of both. I think a lot of traditional Pakistani people would probably view me as very English, but sometimes also English people say to me "You're English, not Pakistani" and I say "No, I'm Pakistani" because I see that differently. ... The problem is sometimes that the religion and the culture are very intermeshed and if you're not religious that can be difficult'.

Finally Shadi, who is quadrilingual in Farsi, French, Swedish and English, and whose family fled Iran after the Iranian Revolution, says: *'You become rootless, don't you? ... I don't feel English or Swedish at all. I don't miss Sweden; I only miss my family there. In France I feel very much at home. If I had the chance to move to France I would. I was very close to my grandfather and grandmother and my grandfather spoke of how much he loved France and all his memories as a student in France. Paris – that's where I feel the happiest. And Iran, I feel very proud ... very Iranian but it's also very sorrowful. It's tied to a lot of suffering and pain. So I am not proud of being Iranian today, I'm proud of being Persian, which is different. I am proud of the Iranian culture before and I try to give that to my children. But when I go to Iran, I don't feel at home ... I wouldn't go to Iran without my husband or my parents – I feel very insecure. ... My parents raised me very much to be an Iranian – there was no doubt – I was an Iranian being raised in England, so I always knew who I was. It's benefited me – English and Swedish were just additional languages ... I don't know much about the English culture. ..Iranian and French are very similar in our traditions and culture and the way we are ... there's no culture clash ... it's all very similar ... which is also probably why I feel very at home in France'.*

Different Behaviours

Linked to the issue of identity, we were interested to find out whether any of our interviewees felt that they behaved differently depending on which language they are speaking at the time. About one third of those we interviewed mentioned this issue of behaving differently, or were aware that the way that they would normally behave based on one language and culture is not or would not be appropriate in another language community. Clearly this is only likely to arise where there are significant cultural differences as well as linguistic ones between the different communities involved. Thus when asked about this, Saad responded that there are few significant differences in body language or behaviour between Kurds and Arabic speakers in Iraq. The differences that interviewees did notice can be divided into three. The most common was the cultural difference in terms of respect for elders in many non-Western cultures. This was true about Bindi and Pari who were both Gujarati speakers. Pari feels that she is less casual when speaking in Gujarati, more reserved, and puts more thought into what she says, partly because of the cultural environment, whereby elders are respected. Aimee from Togo, who grew up speaking French and Kabye, also mentioned this. When asked if she behaves differently depending on what language she is speaking, she says that she does because she uses Kabye to address elders and part of her culture is that you have to speak respectfully to them. It is unacceptable, for example, to speak to someone older whilst doing something else at the same time.

Vera W also noticed this, but she also notes that Chinese people are more reserved than English people. Vera feels that she is more formal when she speaks Cantonese. This would be particularly true when speaking to elder people where the Cantonese would use more respectful language. She has noticed that Chinese people do not easily express their emotions and she wonders whether she would have had a more open and honest relationship with her parents if she had been raised in a different culture.

For others, though, English was the more reserved language, and they were more expressive when speaking other languages; so Emilio (Spanish and English) uses more body language when speaking Spanish, and Fatima says that the body language she uses with Arabic is different from English in that she uses more gestures and is much more likely to touch people when she is speaking Arabic. She says that this is not to do with the person she is speaking to – if she was speaking to someone bilingual in English and switched to Arabic, her gestures would change and she would be much more likely to touch them.

Parvati said that she uses different intonation, gestures and body language depending on whether she is speaking Hindi or English. She feels that Hindi is a much more expressive language, and that she uses more facial expressions and hand gestures when speaking it. (For example, Parvati said that if she was filmed speaking the two languages and her boyfriend saw the film with the sound turned off, he would be able to tell which language she was speaking from her body language.)

Two interviewees' families noticed a difference in behaviour, although this was hard for the interviewees to pin down. Armelle's Argentinean husband: *'has told me "when you are with your French friends you act differently"'*. In Shadi's case, it is her children who say: *'"When you speak in French you become very French". They say I am much bubblier and happier when I speak French'*.

In three cases, interviewees were aware of a difference in the acceptable levels of directness/tact or in being forthright and loud rather than more softly spoken. Two of these cases concerned the relatively loud and upfront social style that is acceptable in the United States. So Ingrid is aware of the cultural differences in terms of behaviour in the United States and in Sweden, and she is aware that she behaves differently in each context and therefore also in each language: *'In the States it very acceptable to be loud, outspoken. Sweden is not like that'*. Note though that, for Ingrid, this switch occurs when she switches country and not when she switches language – unlike all of the above examples. In another example an interviewee with a mixed-language American and French background was identified as a foreigner in the United States, although she has no accent and she feels that the only difference was that she was more softly spoken and less aggressive than the typical American-English speaker.

In Helen's case, growing up in Holland, she is aware of a noticeable difference in terms of tactfulness/directness between English and Dutch culture. Perhaps because of her English father's influence she considers herself less direct than the average Dutch person, but she still noticed that in England conversations were much less direct or less blunt. Initially this caused her some problems: *'Dutch is a bit more of a rough language and Dutch people are straightforward and to the point. And sometimes, with colleagues, [in England] they can think "What are you saying?" Because they are used to you going round and round the point. Here I am seen as quite direct, whereas for a Dutch person I am quite a softy. It is quite difficult because I don't intend to be rude but [in England] I can be seen as rude because of being very direct'.*

Conclusion

It is not at all surprising that interviewees reported that they behaved differently when speaking different languages (or at least when they were in different cultural contexts). I wondered whether this would make anyone feel uncomfortable or hypocritical. I wondered if people might feel that one behaviour was more natural and therefore that one was more artificial. But this was not the case. All those who reported these differences felt completely comfortable with the switching, and some clearly relished the more expressive language and the options that it gave them. It was also clear that some people were blending – they would be at the extreme of behaviour in one culture that was closest to the norm in their other culture. This is reassuring for parents raising children with languages that are linked with cultural communities that have very different norms or ways of behaving. It seems that children will learn the two behaviours in exactly the same way as they learn the two languages, and this will feel completely natural and normal to them and not at all uncomfortable.

Many interviewees had come to terms with their identities. Some had done so by choosing one side. Some sided with the majority language and culture where they lived. Some clearly had a strong ethnic minority identity. Some were comfortable being a mixture of several things, and some felt that 'being simultaneously insiders and outsiders' was a distinct advantage. Some were pleased to stand out and were proud to be different. Others, though, clearly did feel uncomfortable about not being easily able to fit themselves into any one box. It is very difficult to identify any one particular factor that links with feeling comfortable or uncomfortable on this point. Both those who are comfortable, and those who are not, included interviewees in mixed-language families and migrant children, both those with monolingual and multilingual parents, children who experienced racism and those who did not, children who moved several times and those who did not, children who were speaking very marginalised languages, children speaking perceived high-status languages, and those who were religious and those who were not. In several cases, interviewees said that they identified with one community even if it was not now or had not been for a long time their strongest language or the language that they used most regularly. Several of the interviewees described feeling that they were different from other people where they grew up, and concluded that they really belonged to somewhere that their minority language was spoken, only to visit there as young adults and discover that they did not fit in there either. Claudia, who could easily have been forgiven for feeling somewhat rootless as a result of having lived in six different countries during her diplomatic childhood, is one of the small number of interviewees who have a clear and singular identity. Similarly, Mohammed's views are both very well thought through and very positive, despite significant overt racism and some other facets of his bilingual childhood not being ideal (e.g. his experience at a Saturday language school).

The views expressed above show that identity may be a concern to bilingual children that lingers and leaves a legacy for adults – this is also supported by the scientific literature.

- One simple answer is to pick one side or other as the primary identity for your children; although clearly several of our interviewees did not follow the wishes of their parents on this point, the ability to visit and the perceived status of each language or community may be important here.
- A more complex strategy, but one that might pay dividends in the long term, is to clearly build opportunities to create pride in two or more heritages. This is easier for those juggling two languages of equally developed countries that are similar. Families who are refugees who have a very mixed experience and relationship with their home country may have a particular difficulty here. As parents we may all be tempted in conversations between adults to criticise government decisions or lack of progress on certain points, and perhaps we should be very careful to temper these as children get older and can understand more with conversations that convey respect for a culture and celebrate cultural events.
- Finally, several interviewees mentioned being raised to be 'proud to be different', and some who had not been raised in this way were raising their own children with this ethos. Some children, due to their personality, may take to this more easily than others, but this might be a useful point to stress whatever other strategies are adopted.

23 Studying and Working Abroad as Young Adults, Choosing Where to Live More Permanently and Using Bilingualism at Work

It seems striking to us that around a quarter of our interviewees elected to go abroad and study or work in a country where their minority language was spoken as a majority language when they were around 17 or 18 years old. Another six interviewees lived and worked or studied in a country speaking a relevant language when they were young adults. In some of these cases, the interviewees had already visited the country for holidays during their childhoods, but for others this was the first experience of speaking what had been for them a minority language in a place where this was the common or majority language.

For some interviewees, this was an important part of reclaiming a language that they had not always been comfortable speaking. Charles, whose mother had spoken Dutch to him as a child but stopped after a while, did his first degree in the UK and then went to Holland to do his Masters and PhD, which were both in English. He was embarrassed about speaking Dutch because he did not want to make mistakes. As he did not have much interaction with Dutch people on a day-to-day basis before his arrival in Holland, his Dutch was basic. When he started living in Holland his Dutch became much better, and by the time he left his Dutch had improved considerably, and he felt more comfortable speaking it. He was discussing research topics with his colleagues in Dutch, which also taught him how to express more complex ideas in this language. Socially, he spoke to his Dutch colleagues in Dutch. Charles also explained to us why he wanted to go to Holland: *'One of the reasons why I went to Holland to do my Masters and PhD was to get in touch with my Dutch side, but on arrival I realised that I have no Dutch side [laughs]!'*. You will have noted that this echoes the comments of several interviewees above about identity, whereby they expected to feel more at home or more at one with their minority-language identity by moving to a country that spoke that language. Often this experience, as with Charles, instead confirmed that their identity was more closely tied up with the country that they had grown up in (or that they did not feel that they fully belonged in either place).

These visits were particularly common amongst the interviewees who had preferred not to reply to their parents speaking a minority language (i.e. those described in the section titled 'resistance', from p.81 onwards). In fact, all four of the interviewees who consistently refused to respond to their parents in one of their languages throughout their childhoods travelled to live and work or study in a country where that language was the majority language as young adults. Although none of them suggest the resistance (or issues linked to it) in some way provided the motivation for them to make the move, Ingrid, Helen and Armelle explicitly make the link between these trips abroad and the eventual end of their resistance as adults. Ingrid told us that: *'It was not until I was 16 and I went to study in the States that I started to speak English back to [my mother]'*. Spanish, French and Italian-speaking Armelle returned from Europe to Argentina to study when she was 19, and this eventually led her to respond to her mother in Spanish, whereas she had mainly responded in French until then. Helen (who was raised hearing Dutch and English but who preferred to respond in Dutch only) came to the UK to do a degree, which led her to talk to her English father in English also for the first time (but only when they are in England).

In some cases, such visits seem to have been critical in interviewees retaining a language as adults. Emilio, who had learnt his English entirely through his school and who spoke Spanish at home and in the community, had the opportunity to go to the United States for eight weeks when he was 18. Here he was immersed in English and worked for a company owned by a family friend and felt that, for him, this was a breakthrough because he had never been in an English-speaking environment before. Some years later, Emilio went to the UK to study for an MA. He says that he literally did not speak a word of Spanish for several months, and this really helped to cement his English. Emilio estimated that only around half of the students in his (bilingual English/ Spanish) class can still speak English today. Certainly I got a sense speaking to him that had it not been for these trips out of Argentina to anglophone countries, Emilio might also have gradually lost much of the English that he learnt at school.

In Bindi's case (having lived in Kenya and the UK and having spoken English at school in both places and a mixture of English and Gujarati at home), she went to the Gujarat region of India when she was 22. This was her first ever visit to India: *'I stayed three months and I was working in the villages so I had to speak Gujarati. My Gujarati improved from everyday Gujarati to quite complicated discussions around politics and economics and things like that ... to the point where I could hold my own in a discussion. So I picked up vocabulary and terminology that I had never heard of before, because it wasn't used at home. And at that moment I felt "I can do this in Gujarati and I can do it in English". And that was a proud moment'*. Bindi noticed one issue when she was in India where she realised that she used words that the Gujarati community in Mombasa has borrowed from Swahili, which they now consider to be normal Gujarati, but which no one in Gujarat recognised or understood. (For another example of this, see p.33 for Matilde's account of how she only noticed that the family were mixing Swahili into their Italian sentences when they returned from Africa to Italy.)

Pedro found the same thing when he lived for two years in Spain as an adult, having grown up in bilingual and segregated Texas. He noticed differences between the Spanish used in Texas and the Spanish used in Spain. He also had a problem with mixing languages. As someone whose family mixed Spanish and English a lot at home, he found that he would forget words in Spanish and struggle to find the words he needed when he could not add an English word if he sometimes needed to.

Vera W went with her mother to visit China. Although this was only for a holiday, the visit clearly made a deep impression on her. The village her mother had grown up in had been flooded when a dam was built, and her grandmother's gravestone and their old house were under water. Most of the village had moved away from China. Vera's mother did not enjoy her visit back to China. However, Vera was much more positive: *'I went back to China and I found it very comforting. I felt really comfortable there. It was very beautiful and peaceful. I understood where my mother was coming from. I saw the hardships my family had gone through ... still go through. It was pretty primitive ... I also saw what communism had done to certain families ... My mother wouldn't even sleep in the village, we had to go back to the town and stay in a western apartment'.* Vera says that she would like to return to China and study more there – but as a Cantonese speaker she realises that today Mandarin is essential in China, and that she would need to learn to speak Mandarin.

Choosing Where to Live More Permanently

Just under half of the interviewees were living in a country speaking the language that was the majority language when they were growing up, and in most cases this was the same country where they had grown up. Ten interviewees had moved to live in a country where their minority language as a child was the majority language, and eight interviewees were living in countries speaking an entirely new language. Where interviewees had moved countries, there were often, no doubt, economic, academic or other reasons for these moves (one interviewee moved as a refugee as an adult). Some interviewees mentioned that they would actually prefer to be living somewhere else.

Only a few interviewees explained the reasons behind their decision to live somewhere particular. One that did so was Armelle, who explained: *'When I finished university, I had a crisis because my family were off around the world and I asked myself what I was doing in Argentina. I had the opportunity to move back to Paris and I packed my suitcase and decided to go back to France. ... At some point you start to think "Where do I want to be ... where do I belong in France or in Argentina?" But then I decided to move back to Argentina – I chose Argentina because I am close to my extended family there. In Argentina I miss the culture in France but Argentina is very emotional and warm, whereas I feel that my French [extended] family is colder'.* This is striking as, in terms of identity, Armelle explains that she feels more French than Argentinean (see p.166).

Markus was the only interviewee who explicitly said that he had moved countries for reasons linked to a language preference. He told us that he moved from Germany to the UK in 2000 in order to study, citing the fact that he liked speaking English as one of the reasons he decided to leave Germany.

Conversely, several interviewees said that the majority language where they live determined the amount of a language they were using. So Marion, who lives in England for career reasons, said: *'If we were living in Wales I would be speaking Welsh a lot more and I would be doing everything in Welsh'.*

Work

Out of our more than 40 interviewees, only two (Saad and Velji) were working as translators or interpreters, and in both cases, these were second careers as both had initially trained and/or worked in another career. Velji translates between the languages he learnt as a child, whereas Saad translates from either Kurdish or Arabic (the two languages he learnt as a child) into English, which he learnt as a foreign language at school and after he moved to the UK, and vice versa. Two more interviewees had worked as interpreters or translators to help pay their way through university or as a first job when moving to a new country before they moved on to their preferred career. Some interviewees had studied languages at university but had then gone on to other careers. Some interviewees told us that they had been expected to have a career involving languages but had resisted, so Sylvia said: *'There is a danger of allowing the [bilingual] gift to rule one's life. There can be huge pressure to make bilingualism the keystone of career decisions. Being a lawyer is far more interesting (and better paid) than being a translator!'*

However, despite not having followed careers as a linguist per se, many other interviewees were using their languages at work – whether as advice workers, therapists, lawyers, or aid workers. In some cases, they were in jobs that required a particular additional language, while in others their languages were a bonus that they could use but which their colleagues would not have. Several other interviewees mentioned that their languages had helped them find work when they started out, or had meant that they got higher-paid jobs than they would have done otherwise. Claudia said she had walked into a well-paid job in the City because she spoke German. She also worked as a bilingual secretary and *'got paid a fortune'*. Sabina told us that speaking Urdu: *'helped me, for example, to switch careers when I was really fed up with my job. It helped me change direction. I quite enjoyed being able to use it and to help people from my culture or community. Several of my jobs have been language posts [i.e. speaking Urdu was a requirement]'.*

Velji explained that the fact that he spoke three or four languages fluently had opened up a lot of career opportunities for him in his first career with BAT. Parallel to his normal role, because of his languages, he was initially used as an interpreter for some training, but ended up running subsequent training sessions and becoming the primary trainer. This in turn led to many new opportunities for him for advancement within the company.

Armelle, who works setting up and running international conferences, felt that her three fluent languages have helped her a great deal in her career. She has often been asked about them or asked questions in these languages at interviews, and she is sure that they have helped her get jobs in the best companies in her field.

Marion, the Welsh/English bilingual who had such trouble learning to read at her school in London and who is now a professor of English literature, commented that: *'Learning to read in Welsh paid off considerably in later years when I wrote a book on the Arthurian legends, Women in Arthurian Literature. I did a chapter on Lady Charlotte Guest who translated the Mabinogion [a collection of Welsh folk tales] and I could look at her translations and compare it to the Mabinogion because I could read it in Welsh'.*

Altogether, 25 interviewees mentioned that their bilingualism had helped them at some point in their careers, work or studies.

Conclusion

Although ours is not a scientific sample, it does seem clear that being bilingual has helped a lot of our interviewees in their post-school studies or in their careers. It also seems clear that those people we interviewed were more likely than the average person to have lived and worked abroad and/or to have moved or settled in a new country. Very few of the interviewees in our sample had jobs directly revolving around their languages, but most were able to use their languages at work as a bonus or a helpful but not determining factor in their work.

- Do not be surprised if young adults who have been raised bilingually decide to travel to a country where what has been a minority language for them is widely spoken. This may well be part of a process of finding out 'where they really belong'. If our sample is typical they may be hoping to find a simple way of belonging more completely in one place but, in fact, will often come away after such a trip understanding that their identity is more complex.
- Do not expect those who have been raised bilingually to necessarily end up in careers that revolve around languages. Many will find ways to use their languages at work but very few will be translators, interpreters, or language teachers.

24 Relationships

Marriages and Partnerships

Of our 40 or so interviewees, 30 were either married or were in long-term relationships. I wondered whether adults raised bilingually would choose to have a relationship in the stronger of their two languages. Alternatively, I wondered if they would have a relationship with someone who spoke the language that they most identified with or within the language community that they felt that they belonged to. Although some did, there were enough exceptions to make it clear that there are no simple correlations here. We asked some questions about the first languages of each of a couple, but we also asked about the language that they use to speak to each other, as these were by no means always the same.

The 30 interviewees who are now married or in long-term relationships divide exactly into three groups of ten. Ten of our interviewees had partners or spouses whose first language was one that the interviewee had never spoken whilst growing up. Ten interviewees were in a relationship with someone who spoke their childhood majority language. So Camilla, who grew up hearing Danish at home and English in the community and at school in England, is married to an Englishman. Ingrid, who grew up hearing English at home and Swedish in the community and at school, married a Swedish man (although they now live in London). The remaining ten interviewees were in a relationship with someone who spoke their childhood minority language. (This includes some who are also married to bilinguals in the same languages. So Bindi, who spoke Gujarati and English at home and English at school in both Kenya and London, is married to another bilingual English/Gujarati speaker.)

It was also clear that in many cases the relative strength of two or more languages did not have an impact on the language of someone's long-term partner or spouse. Tom married a Croatian woman, although he feels that his English is the stronger of his two languages. Neither did the interviewees' stronger identity necessarily have an impact – Marion married a monolingual English speaker although she identified as being Welsh.

Parvati is currently teaching her (English) boyfriend to speak Hindi. This is partly for pragmatic reasons as they may work in India in the future, but also because she wants him to be able to understand the other world view that she has. Parvati feels that Hindi is a more romantic language. She is aware that she uses Hindi more often when she is angry (as her mother did). She is also aware that she uses different intonation, gestures and body language. She feels that Hindi is a much more expressive language, and that she uses more facial expressions and hand gestures when speaking it. Hence perhaps it is important to her that her boyfriend understands some of the language.

Other interviewees also talked interestingly about the use of languages within their social relationships (whether with friends or as couples). So Claudia said that, despite her Brazilian partner, *'All of my social network, all of my current friends speak German, are half German. . . . I find it easier to speak to someone who is bilingual because I can throw the odd German word in'.*

Sarah's last long-term partner was German, and her brother's first long-term girlfriend was also German, which made her mother very happy *'like she was given a trophy!'* Sarah feels this sent a symbolic message to her mother: *'You have succeeded in what you've been doing all these years. . .'.* During this relationship, Sarah's German improved greatly and she started to express emotions and 'things of the heart' in German a lot more, although her partner understood English as well. He tried to speak to her in English because this was her preferred language, so they tried to accommodate each other all the time. She would express more complex emotions in English. During this phase she started to switch between languages with much more ease: *'The more I speak it the more likely it is that I will continue to speak it; it lubricates the tongue and makes it easier'.*

Changes in Languages Used with Parents Over Time

Several interviewees mentioned that the language pattern that was established between themselves and their parents changed after they reached adulthood. In several different sections we have described how difficult it seems to be for family members to change the language that they speak to one another. However, once children have left home and families no longer live together and interact on a daily basis, some interviewees found changing the language of a relationship much more possible – in some cases these were deliberate choices from either the parent or the child. In others, the changes were not sought and just happened naturally. Having a break, including – in some cases – a change of country and context may mean that it is easier to change the language of a relationship. We have described above how Armelle, Helen and Ingrid all started to reply to their parents in a language that they had hitherto been reluctant to speak after they left home (and in all three cases moved country to where the language they had been reluctant to speak was the majority language). But other families also made changes without any move. Sometimes this was the initiative of the interviewee, so when she was in her mid-20s, for instance, Sabina made a conscious decision that she would speak Urdu to her father as she really wanted to maintain and improve her Urdu. In Tom's case, he and his father seem to have switched languages. Originally, Tom's father would speak Croatian and Tom would reply in English. Now, Tom speaks to his father more in Croatian than English, but says that his father *'probably speaks to me more in English than in Croatian!'* The shift on Tom's side may have followed his marriage to a Croatian woman and their decision to raise their children bilingually speaking Croatian and English. On Tom's father's side, one wonders if he has simply gained better English and developed a habit of speaking more English through his years of living in Australia.

In some cases, the interviewees implied that their parents had adopted speaking a particular language to help the interviewee as a child gain a command of that language, but felt that they no longer needed to do so once the child had grown up. Zwelibanzi said that his father spoke English to him so he would be fluent in the language, which would help him at school and in his career, but now, since Zwelibanzi lives in England, his father speaks to him in Zulu as: *'There is no need for him to speak in English'.*

Astrid had spoken only English with her German parents who had moved from Germany to Australia when aged 12 and 19. They had decided to speak English to their children to help them to integrate. After Astrid had left home, her parents moved back to Germany, and from then on the language that she used with them shifted partially to German. Nowadays she speaks more and more German with them when in Germany, and they would reply mostly in German, especially her mother. However, Astrid also acknowledged: *'If I've been in Germany and I come back to London and I'm speaking to my mum on the phone I'm still in a German mode and I may just keep speaking German with her, but you always go back to English'.*

Markus's experience is interesting as he was one of the families that had the fewest rules, where his parents spoke both languages and these were freely mixed within sentences. Nowadays Markus's mother only speaks English to him, and this has already been the case for a long time (probably since the early 1990s). Sometimes she tries to speak German to him, out of habit since she lives in Germany and speaks German all the time in her day-to-day life, but Markus generally refuses to speak German with her.

Christopher is in his late sixties and he has also noticed a change in the language he uses to speak to his French mother, who has now lived in the UK for 70 years. This seems to be connected to a change in roles that is perhaps linked to his mother's increasing age and some loss of memory. Until recently Christopher would always speak French to her, but then he started to switch into English. *'Consciously, that's something that's happening more and more. When she speaks in French I answer back in English . . . I'm growing up, I suppose, becoming independent! [laughs]. . . There are times when I speak French to her, but it becomes much more a deliberate thing. What I want to say to her is best said in French and French language can carry the meanings, or I want to create a rapport'.* As she is losing her memory, Christopher has to be more deliberate with language use when he speaks to her. *'If I'm pushed and I want to make sure she gets the meaning, then I will speak deliberately in French. She's never become English. I suppose it's natural that I go back to her roots rather than what I prefer to do'.*

Some interviewees now speak a mixture of their two languages to their parents – but they still reflected very thoughtfully on why they spoke particular languages on different occasions. Ingrid told us: *'I know with my mum sometimes, if I get really frustrated or angry, I'll sometimes say things in Swedish, just because that seems like an angrier language. . . . If I want to be stern with her, I'll sometimes switch to Swedish. With my husband although we speak mostly Swedish, I will sometimes throw in the odd word in English. . . . I also think that it is power in a way to have these languages. So when I get angry with my mother and I chose to speak Swedish it's also because it gives me an edge because I speak Swedish better than her'.*

However, other interviewees told us that that they would like to switch the language that they speak with their parents – usually because they now have fewer opportunities to speak one language and want to keep using it. So Claudia now lives and works in England, and she uses English a lot more than German now. She makes an effort to speak German with her family. Despite this, sticking to long-established patterns, her mother will reply to her in English – causing Claudia to switch back to English, which is now her stronger language. She also says: *'It's funny that I tend to speak German with my family when it's something serious. When it's something frivolous, I tend to do it in English. . . . German feels more . . . I don't know . . . serious'.*

There was also one example of a parent maintaining opposition to a child's language choice well into adult life. You may remember that Snjezana's elder sister taught her to speak Esperanto in spite of quite strong opposition from their parents. Snjezana still speaks Esperanto with her husband and says: *'My mother still gets very annoyed about this. She thinks it is a waste of time. She feels that it is a wasted opportunity. She feels that if we spoke other languages it would contribute to our fluency in those languages . . . and she feels annoyed because she feels excluded as well'.*

Sisters and Brothers

Several interviewees mentioned using occasional or particular phrases from a language with their siblings even when they primarily communicate in another language. In some cases, this just seemed to be an established family usage, which the children continued. So Charles speaks French to his brothers, but sometimes they use a Dutch word for a particular thing, like a 'windowsill': *'For some reason a "windowsill" for us is always going to be a "vensterbank"'.*

However, for some of the interviewees, the use of a common (almost private) language seems to bring them closer together or to be more natural. So, for Zwelibanzi, who grew up speaking Zulu and English and now lives in England, he has siblings in the UK, and generally they speak in English, but when discussing family issues Zwelibanzi speaks to them in Zulu. *'It comes naturally. . . . If it is something emotional, or I want to emphasise something to my brother, I find myself speaking in Zulu, because those thoughts you can't express them in English, you prefer to express them in your own language to be more effective'.*

Parvati described continuing to speak Hindi with her sister when her mother (who was their main input in Hindi) moved 200 miles away to work during the week when Parvati was 11 years old. This meant that the input in Hindi for Parvati and her sister was reduced but they continued to speak Hindi together – mainly because there were things that could be said in Hindi that had no English equivalents: *'There are these wonderful expressive phrases . . . in Hindi there's this phrase "Which radish field are you from?" If you use this in an argument, it's hilarious, it's impossible to stay angry because it's not insulting but at the same time it's so insulting. English doesn't have that kind of layering . . . richness'.*

One interviewee describes that it is still difficult for her to change the language that she speaks with her brother. Armelle still speaks French to her brother, even though they are both living in Argentina. When Armelle, her husband and her brother meet, Armelle speaks in French to her brother, even though she knows that her husband does not speak much French and she knows that it would be more sensible to speak in Spanish, which everyone could understand. But she finds it difficult to change the language of this relationship. It just feels very unnatural to her. (Admittedly, as I mentioned above, the fact that her brother has told her 'that he likes me more in French than in Spanish' may not help with this!)

For one interviewee, Markus, the choice of language with his brother had been slightly awkward: 'With my brother, recently I have started speaking English to him again but usually it has been German. He has just spent six months in the US and so his English has improved and he is less reluctant to speak English. For the last 5–6 years it has been a bit awkward. We never really knew which language we should speak to each other. We would start in English and switch to German and then switch back to English. I kind of feel that I should speak German to him and he probably kind of feels that he should speak English to me'.

Families Without a Single Fluent Common Language

Some families ended up without one common language that everyone could speak confidently and comfortably. This can occur with mixed marriages and extended families, so, as mentioned above, one of our interviewees, Josune, was raised speaking Basque and Spanish and is married to a Czech man. Within the nuclear family the common language is English. When they visit Josune's family who do not speak English, there is no common language between her family and her husband. This did not surprise me. What I did find more surprising were the families where there is no one common language even within the nuclear family (i.e. the parents and their children). This only occurred in three families, all migrants. In one family the children migrated relatively late, and one other example of this concerns the family where the mother had a serious mental health problem, which clearly impacted heavily on many facets of family life.

Fatima's parents had left Morocco to come to the UK to work as a chef, and their children joined them when Fatima was 10 years old. Fatima's parents had not been educated in Morocco and did not learn English. Fatima has four brothers and one sister. Her eldest brother was 18 when he came to the UK, and her youngest brother was born there. Fatima's eldest brother also never learnt to speak English with any real degree of fluency – although he understands a lot. Fatima's youngest brother who was born in the UK now really prefers to speak English, although again he understands a lot of Arabic, which he can speak, but he is not really comfortable expressing anything complex in the language and will quickly switch back to English. This makes language choice complicated when the family gets together. Her father, mother and eldest brother speak Arabic and might understand some English but do not speak it well. As well as her youngest brother who prefers English, she now has sisters-in-law who do not speak Arabic. This means that the middle siblings do spend some time translating from Arabic to English, and from English to Arabic when all of the family gets together. Fatima herself tends to speak Arabic to all of her older brothers, but English to her younger sister and brother.

The second example is Mumtaz. Mumtaz's family had moved from Pakistan to the UK when Mumtaz was seven. Although Mumtaz's father spoke and understood a little English, Mumtaz's mother did not. Mumtaz acted as the main carer for her family during her mother's mental illness, which lasted for between three and four years from when Mumtaz was about 10 years old. Mumtaz's father was working nights at this time. Mumtaz generally preferred to speak English to her younger brothers and sisters to avoid saying something that might set her mother off if she overheard it. Mumtaz believes that, in many ways, her younger brothers and sister who were born in the UK had life easier than she did because she and her sister would speak English to them at home, so that they had some knowledge of English before they started school. However, these younger siblings are not confident speaking Urdu and much prefer speaking English today. If they speak to their parents in Urdu/Punjabi they will include English words and her youngest brother, who is 21, will say: *'How do I say that? How can I explain that to Mum?'* This means that in Mumtaz's family, there is no single common language that everyone feels very confident speaking. In contrast to her siblings, Mumtaz's Urdu is much better, and she does not use English words.

The final, and particularly poignant, case is that of Antony, who thinks he has lost out by being not fully bilingual because his Greek was limited, and therefore he could not express everything he wanted to say to his mum. He feels that his Greek started to become limited very soon after he started primary school aged around six or seven. During his mum's funeral, he was to give a eulogy. He asked the priest in which language he should do this. The priest's advice was to do it in whichever language or way that would most 'come from his heart'. He decided to do the speech in English. He now regrets this as, assuming that there is an afterlife, he realises that his mother may not have been able to understand what he was saying about her. He felt sad about this afterwards.

Only the last of these interviewees mentioned this as a downside or disadvantage of being bilingual. Both Fatima and Mumtaz's families had faced serious challenges. Both also regretted that their parents had not learnt more English. Mumtaz's case is clearly more severe and, in this case because of her mother's ill health, the children may have formed almost as strong a bond with Mumtaz herself as the oldest child as they did with their mother. In Fatima's case, the fact that her parents had never been educated in Morocco was probably a problem that inhibited them from learning English once in the UK. In Antony's case, perhaps it was the very formal and public setting of a funeral that put him off speaking Greek, which he was less confident speaking although he was still using it with his mother at home up until this point. Nonetheless, it does seem to us both surprising and quite problematic to have this minority of examples of multilingual families where relationships seem fractured by language in this way in the long term.

Conclusion

Given the struggles that many couples had in changing the language of their relationship, it was surprising to note the degree and number of changes between interviewees and their parents as adults. Clearly the fact that parents and their adult children often do not live together, and so there are many long breaks in which to seek to change habits, may help.

Having two languages may give siblings more options in their uses of language. Generally this was seen as positive. Switching to a home language can convey intimacy and emotional closeness, for example, or it can be helpful in distinguishing serious from more informal or humorous conversations. Only one interviewee reported the fact that their two brothers had different preferred languages had introduced some awkwardness into their relationship.

- The families who had no common language within the same generation worried me much more. If you migrate to a new country and raise your children with a home-language/majority-language system, work hard to ensure that your children do retain the home languages through their teens. An alternative is to accept that you will need to gain a very good knowledge of the majority language so as to be able to speak this to your children. Even then, as with Ingrid, unless you are very talented, your children – as native speakers – may always have a better mastery of the majority language than you.
- Provided that family members can understand the languages well, consider adopting the system used by Armelle's parents whereby each person <u>speaks</u> in the language they are most confident in and others reply in a different language (it is surprising to us that this seems to be so rare).

25 Raising Children Monolingually or Bilingually and the Reasons Given

Although all of the interviewees felt glad that they had been raised bilingually, I wondered which languages they would choose to speak to their own children and how many of them would decide to raise their own children bilingually. Of our interviewees, 29 had children.

Language Choices with Children

Firstly I wondered whether interviewees raised with one language at home and another in the community would be more likely to speak to their children in the language that they were 'mothered' or parented in, even if this was not necessarily their strongest language. Almost half of the interviewees where this choice applies speak to their children in a language that neither of their parents used to speak to them – normally their childhood majority language. So Antony spoke Greek at home, Pari spoke Gujarati at home and Camilla's parents spoke Danish to her at home, but all are raising their children in English. Similarly, Aimee speaks French to her child, although French was Aimee's school and majority language, whereas she spoke Kabye at home.

In some cases, choosing not to speak a home language was done explicitly to achieve a bilingual outcome for an interviewee's child; so, for example, Tom and his wife speak English and Croatian to their son respectively because Tom's wife's Croatian is stronger than her English (which was learnt at school/as an adult) and they wanted to use the 'one person, one language' approach. This means that Tom speaks to his son in English, which he learnt only from age 12 and which his parents never spoke to him when he was a child (but which he feels is the stronger of his two languages).

Only one interviewee specifically referred to this issue. Sylvia (raised speaking English at home and French in the community and at school) told us that she originally started to try to raise her children bilingually, but that it felt too unnatural when she tried to speak French to her children: '... it also felt very artificial ...I had been mothered in English. I felt like I was pretending to be a phony French mother, I was pretending to be someone I wasn't'. However, this was the only opinion given on this issue, and no one else who took this route seems to have had any problem at all.

I also wondered if interviewees would always speak to their children in the language of the community that they identified most strongly with. This was also not the case, and there was a fairly even divide between the interviewees on this. In the section on identity above (on p.165), we mentioned that only seven interviewees said clearly that they felt that they belonged to one community more than the other. Of these, five had children, and three of these do speak the language they identified with to their children (Armelle in French, Josune in Basque, and Sylvia in English) whereas two do not (Zwelibanzi identified with Zulu but speaks English to his children, and Marion identified with Welsh but speaks English to hers).

In fact, it seems to me that our interviewees mostly selected their strongest and most current language as the language to speak to their children regardless of where or how they had learnt it. Many interviewees were more or less balanced bilinguals where there was not a clearly stronger or weaker language. Of the 11 interviewees who were parents for whom we could identify a relatively strong and a relatively weak language, eight had decided to speak to their children in the stronger language and only three had chosen the weaker one. One (borderline but interesting) example in this last group of three who chose to speak what seems to be, for her, her second language to their children is Mumtaz, who chose to speak English to her children which was her community and school language, whereas she heard and spoke exclusively Urdu until she left Pakistan when she was seven and after that her parents continued to speak Urdu to her at home, although she herself increasingly used English. To the interviewer, Mumtaz's English was indistinguishable from a native speaker, with a London accent and phraseology, except that Mumtaz herself said: *'Even now, when I think, I think in my language [Urdu/ Punjabi] in my mind and then I translate it into English'*. It surprised us, given this comment, that Mumtaz had decided to speak English and not Urdu/Punjabi to her children. However, Mumtaz was also the child who looked after her younger siblings extensively whilst her mother was unwell and most of this 'mothering' of her siblings was done in English. So it is possible that the fact that she had already established a role of parenting in English may have influenced her decision. Another example is Sabina, who of her languages said: *'I think in terms of the language and fluency, English is far more dominant, my thinking is in English . . .',* but she has decided to raise her son speaking Urdu (her home language). Another exception to the general finding that interviewees as parents were more likely to speak their strongest language to their children is Astrid, who learnt German solely from a six-month stay in Germany aged around four and an additional four years at a Saturday language school followed by a degree. Apart from the six-month period in Germany, Astrid's parents never spoke German to her. However, Astrid has decided to raise her son speaking German. Again, for Astrid this is a choice between her son being bilingual or not, as her husband is English: *'I want my son to grow up with the second language. I'm going to try to get a German childminder. I'm doing it for a selfish reason as well. I want to improve my German! I'm going to teach my son and learn that way!'*

In the case of the 10 interviewees who grew up in mixed-language family settings, I wondered whether they would be more likely to speak either the language that their mother used to speak to them, or the language that their father used. (This question arose particularly given that many of our interviewees grew up in an era and/or in settings where the bulk of the childcare was left to the women whilst the men went out to work.) A further question that occurred to us was whether our interviewees who were men would speak the language that their father had spoken to them, and whether women would speak their mother's language. The numbers are very small but we could find no correlations here. Of these 10 mixed-language interviewees, two are discounted as there was no clear distinction in terms of which parent spoke which language to them. This leaves us with eight interviewees, of whom five spoke to their children in the language their father had used to them in their childhoods (three women and two men) and three spoke the language their mother had used (two women and one man).

Finally, I wondered whether our bilingual interviewees who as children had either fleetingly or more deeply wanted to 'fit in' might choose to speak the majority language of the community that they now live in to their children. Of the interviewees with children, one did not have this option because she did not speak the majority language where she was then living fluently. Of the rest, almost exactly half spoke the majority language and half spoke a minority language. However, as noted earlier, if we take the group of interviewees who reported the most heartfelt concerns about 'fitting in' during their childhoods (or had problems linked to the fact that they were seen as being different), they were more likely to speak the majority language to their children (Sylvia, Camilla, Vera W and Marion all live in England and speak English to their children.)

Raising Children Bilingually or Monolingually

Of the 30 interviewees with children, very slightly more (16) were raising them bilingually than were not. There is an unexplained gap or a disjuncture between the fact that all interviewees were glad they were raised bilingually and felt it was advantageous, and the fact that a significant proportion had decided not to raise their children bilingually. Those raising children bilingually included those who had grown up in migrant families, and mixed-language families. It seems to us that the children raised in very difficult circumstances (divorces, deaths and other problems), and those who seemed to find their childhood of bilingualism (or more likely the migrations and sense of being rootless, which links into bilingualism) most disturbing or upsetting, were less likely to raise their children bilingually than our sample more generally. However, some of the children who had the most difficult childhoods still raised their own children bilingually.

Most interviewees who had decided to raise their children bilingually did not feel that they needed to explain this to us. However, those who had decided not to raise their children bilingually often had a clear rationale for their decision. Some now regretted it, although others did not. I will discuss the latter group first. Several interviewees decided that one of their languages was not strong enough for them to raise their children speaking it. So, Camilla decided not to adopt the 'one parent, one language' approach and speak Danish to her children because she did not feel comfortable enough speaking Danish, and had read that you should speak the language that you speak most fluently to your child. She did try to speak some Danish in addition to English with her eldest child, but her son resisted this and told her not to speak 'that other language'. Despite this, her son refers to himself as Danish and is very proud of this. Camilla says that she does regret that her Danish was not 'of a standard that I could *speak it more with my children'.* She asked her parents to speak Danish to her children and, although her father did for a while, her mother refused to and has always spoken English to them.

Antony also said that he felt his Greek was not good enough, but also that it would have felt more artificial. Both he and his (Italian/English-speaking) wife were bilinguals without making a conscious effort – it felt natural at the time – and he thinks it would be less natural, more artificial and more of an effort to raise his children bilingually. Also, he and his wife speak English to each other and neither feels that their minority language is good enough to speak it to their children. When going on holiday to Cyprus or Greece his children cannot speak Greek and they rely on Antony to translate.

Zwelibanzi, who now lives in England and has a choice between speaking English and Zulu, gave priority to English: *'Learn English, because you are in England. When they are older I know they'll come back to our culture. Because I did the same thing, actually'.*

Christopher and his wife have two children, a daughter and a son. He did not speak to them in French during their childhood. *'I was very well aware that it required a lot of focus and work and concentration. I question whether I did the right thing or not. For a language you've got to use it'.* They just picked up the odd word from him. If he was totally French, he thinks he would have probably made the effort. He appreciates the opportunity he has had and thinks it would be nice to pass it on. He thinks he would introduce French back into the family if he has grandchildren. *'Two languages are better than one!'* (It is hard not to wonder whether the fact that his mother left the family when his parents separated when he was 10, and the fact that thereafter Christopher says that he felt closer to his English-speaking father than to his French-speaking mother, also had any influence on this decision.)

Several interviewees' decisions were influenced by their own experiences as children in one way or another. So Marion, for example, who had lived in a family divided between English and Welsh, has two sons with her English husband, but she has not taught them much Welsh. *'I don't want to build up an environment in the way that I grew up where it really divided the family into two'.*

As mentioned above, other interviewees did try to speak a particular language to their children that would have meant that they were raised bilingually but just found that it felt too unnatural. For Sylvia: *'When I had my first child I started trying to speak French to her. Walking round the house with this baby . . . trying to speak French to her. And not only was it somewhat irritating to my husband, jabbering away when he didn't understand. . . . My French identity was strong when I was at school but by then, aged 32, I had been here in England for some time. It was emotionally very, very important to me to be genuine with my family so I decided to stop'.* Clearly, unlike the nine other interviewees who parented in a language that they had not been parented in, Sylvia felt this was very unnatural. We must also bear in mind that, by this time, English was Sylvia's stronger language; as she lives in England it is also the majority language, and as a child Sylvia had been one of the interviewees who raised concerns around 'fitting in'.

Some interviewees just found it difficult to change the language that they had become used to speaking. Although Pedro wishes he had spoken to his second daughter (who is now six) in Spanish from an early age, he did not and now regrets this, but finds it hard to change. He explains that he has not spoken Spanish very much since he left home, and thus it is now habitual for him to speak English and he was not able to break this habit when his daughter was born. *'Since I left home, English is just what I speak, English just comes easier'.*

For others, although they had intended to raise their children bilingually, this just never happened: Pari and her husband who also speaks Gujarati, but who speak English between themselves, did not speak Gujarati to their children. She is not sure why she and her husband did not speak Gujarati to their children, but she says: *'We didn't make a conscious decision not to. The plan was to do it. The longer you leave it the harder it becomes. It just didn't happen'.*

Vera C, who is now 90, married a diplomat and travelled around the world as her husband's postings shifted. Their children went to boarding school back in the UK for much of the time. Vera cannot remember if she ever spoke French to them when they were very young, although she is very positive about bilingual childhoods for her great grandchildren, as one of her granddaughters is married to a Romanian man. Vera told her to *'ask him to speak Romanian to the children'.*

We mentioned earlier that (Urdu and English-speaking) Mumtaz speaks English to her children, as her husband also speaks to them in English (although he does speak Urdu/Punjabi), and the input from Mumtaz's parents has been very important to the children. In spite of only having input from their grandparents, the elder two children speak and understand Urdu/Punjabi well, and while the youngest, a son, has been more resistant, Mumtaz thinks that this may be changing now.

In Adeyinka's case, the fact that his wife does not speak Yoruba has until now prevented him from speaking it to his daughter. He is married to an Igbo speaker. He and his wife communicate in English and they have a one-year-old daughter. Adeyinka would like her to speak Yoruba but he has not started speaking this language to her yet, and he is somewhat inhibited by the fact that his wife does not understand Yoruba.

As with Pedro above, many of those who have not raised their children bilingually now regret this. Daniela is clearest about this. She speaks English and French fluently, as well as some Italian. She has two children: a son, now in his 20s, and a daughter who is eight. She never spoke Italian to her son, who: *'. . .gives me such a hard time because he says: "Why didn't you teach me Italian? I really want to learn Italian now and you never taught me Italian". I didn't feel confident enough with my Italian, that's why'.* Although Daniela's daughter, Jasmine, is already eight, and Daniela has spoken no Italian to her until now, a recent trip to Italy to visit her cousins accompanied by her daughter not only made Daniela want to speak more Italian herself, but has made her decide to try to teach some of the language to her daughter: *'Now I'm quite keen that Jasmine would learn some Italian. She has her second cousin [in Italy] who wants to learn English. My cousin and I are really trying to encourage that friendship. . . .we are trying to get them on Skype so they can try and talk. . . .Jasmine speaks virtually no Italian and her cousin speaks only basic English. When we came back from Italy she was really keen to learn. I bought a Pinocchio puppet and I sometimes play with the puppet and the puppet only speaks Italian, so sometimes in the evening before bed we have these mini conversations. I would say it in Italian and repeat it in English. . . .she likes doing that'.* Now Daniela plans a longer holiday in Italy this summer and she is really looking forward to it. She would like to immerse her daughter in Italian by sending her to an Italian summer camp in Italy with her Italian cousin. She thinks this would help build up their relationship. The visit to Italy made her realise that she had missed this part of her identity a lot, and she now wants her daughter to gain something from it.

Fatima, who had struggled with her transition to school in the UK after moving from Morocco aged 10, said that she felt that it was important that her children could speak enough English to get on well at school, and so she and her husband have both spoken a mix of English and Arabic to her children. *'My worry for my children was that I needed to speak English to them so that they could speak English at school. I thought that if I spoke Arabic to them, that they would find English hard to learn when they went to school and I regretted it . . . especially when I hear . . . you know with the Pakistani community . . .when they come in [to school] and they speak their language fluently. But at the time no one said, "don't do that", and I just thought I was doing the best thing for my kids and I wanted them to start school having English, not having to struggle'.* As a result, her son can speak Arabic and although he has an accent people can understand him. Her daughter can understand a simple sentence but does not actively speak Arabic. When Fatima took her daughter to Morocco after a long break when they had not visited for four years, her daughter cried. She was teased by the other children because she did not speak Arabic and there was also criticism from other family members who felt that her Arabic was not good. Since then, Fatima has made sure that the children visit Morocco every year for at least three weeks, and this has really helped them to get more confident and to speak more Arabic.

Bindi described the decision and the steps that she and her husband took to raise their children bilingually in some detail. Impressively, this also involved a partial change in the language she and her husband used between themselves. Bindi (bilingual English/ Gujarati) is married to a bilingual English and Gujarati speaker and she has two children. Prior to having children she and her husband spoke a mix of English and Gujarati to each other, but when the children were born this changed: *'As an adult, I became very aware that it was very important to be multilingual. And I had these regrets about not learning to read and write in Gujarati. So when we had children both my husband and I made a very conscious decision that my children were going to learn Gujarati. We were living in the USA at this time, so away from community and family. So until my children went to nursery school, probably aged four, they only spoke Gujarati. . . . We spoke exclusively Gujarati in their presence; we made a conscious decision to change the language we spoke between ourselves when the children were there. We had a discussion about it when I was pregnant and we were very particular about it. . . . Our conversations with them at home were only in Gujarati and my mother would come and visit us and sing them nursery rhymes in Gujarati. I also sent them to a Saturday school and they started to learn to read and write in Gujarati but unfortunately the school closed and we haven't found another one close enough. As they get older, it is getting more and more difficult and they are speaking more English. We have decided to stop constantly reminding them, as it feels like nagging [and may be counter productive] and we are hoping that they will come back to it on their own when they are a bit older . . .'.*

Josune is bilingual in Basque and Spanish, her husband speaks a third language (Czech) and the majority language is English, and she felt that she should not try to raise her children quadrilingually, so she felt that she needed to choose between Basque and Spanish. Despite the well-meaning advice from outside that she should speak English or Spanish to them when they were born, she decided to speak Basque. Her family links were crucial in this decision. *'When they were born I did have a conflict [as to] which language I should speak to them. Should it be English, Basque or Spanish? I decided to speak in Basque because I thought that they needed a language which would link them to my family, to be able to feel part of the family. When we have family gatherings I wouldn't want them to feel left out. I also thought that Spanish is so much easier to learn, there are more opportunities to learn Spanish. If I didn't teach them Basque they would never learn it, they would not be able to talk to people, watch TV, feel that they are part of a group, to be able to make friends there'.*

She does not speak any Spanish at home and speaks much less Basque than she used to. Her mother disapproves of her speaking English to the children: *'It hurts me because she doesn't appreciate that I live in a difficult situation here. I have to fight with English and Czech which is their second language'.* She hopes her children will keep it up to be able to get along when they visit family. Her husband was very supportive when she was speaking Basque to the children. He has spoken to them in Czech from birth and that is how she picked the Czech language up. *'If I had more time, I would speak more Basque and Spanish at home "against" English and Czech. It's an uphill struggle with four languages to juggle. My goal is that they manage to communicate and feel that they are attached to that culture and to feel proud of that background. I think I've achieved that. They are proud of speaking Basque. I'm not trying to achieve perfect writing skills. They can learn that later'.*

Two of our interviewees were single parents living in a third language environment and in both cases they felt that they had had to decide between their languages. So Aimee decided to speak French and not Kabye to her daughter, and Christine decided to speak French and not German to hers.

More than half of the 12 interviewees who did not (yet) have children still indicated clear plans to raise their children bilingually or trilingually, although many were already fully aware of some of the challenges involved. For example, Parvati said she would try to raise her own children bilingually. She would like her children to be *'citizens of the world'* rather than a child who feels that they belong to a particular country, and she feels that being bilingual would generally help her children to have wider horizons. Isabelle also said she would try to raise her children bilingually, but added: *'I do think that it's a herculean task though'.* Claudia has some family experience as she has an older brother and sister who both have children, and who both tried to raise them bilingually but have not succeeded. However, she says she would raise her children trilingually – as her partner is Brazilian and they live in England. Despite her own low-key and unpressured bilingual childhood, she is aware that this may not be easy. Not surprisingly, when her nephews and nieces started to drop German and speak more and more English,

Claudia's mother was quite upset about this and started buying them German books and tapes, but to no avail. Claudia mentions that sending her children to a German school would probably be central to success in maintaining their German.

Conclusion

Bilingual parents in our sample have chosen to speak either of their languages to their children. They are speaking home languages, majority languages, languages learnt solely through schooling and never spoken at home, their father's language and their mother's language. A few interviewees mentioned that they felt artificial or unnatural trying to speak a language that their mother or father had not spoken to them, but far more did not notice anything unusual about this. The only correlation that we could find was that bilingual parents who were very concerned about 'fitting in' as children were more likely to speak the majority language where they now live to their children.

- This tells parents just setting out (again) that the only factor determining which of your languages you choose to speak to your child(ren) is that you speak it fluently and well and that you make a clear decision and follow this through consistently.

More than half of the interviewees with children were raising them bilingually. For those that were not, some had tried and failed to do so. Others felt that one of their languages was just not strong enough to do so. Some had just not thought about it until it was too late. Some had believed the myth that speaking the majority language to their children would help with their education. Six, or around half of those who decided not to raise their children bilingually, now regretted this, or felt some sadness even though they feel that they had no real choice. Four interviewees were happy with the decision not to raise children bilingually, and felt that it avoided some problems that they had encountered or that their children would learn the relevant language later.

26 Access to Culture as Adults

A total of 13 interviewees mentioned either the ways that they enjoy reading, music or films or use other resources in both or all their languages (seven interviewees), or the fact that they wished that they could do so more or did not do so in both languages equally (six interviewees). Many of those who wished that they could access more culture in one of their languages talked particularly about reading books.

In some cases, as we have already described (see p.133), the interviewees did not learn to read in all their languages – or only learnt quite late in life and are not confident readers. But Armelle did learn to read both French and Spanish, and says she really enjoyed (and still enjoys) reading books in both languages in the original and not needing to read translations, and she appreciates seeing movies in the original language. She feels that speaking two languages makes you value two cultures and where you come from more. *'Sometimes I feel that I know more about French cinema than my friends who had two French parents, even when I was living in Argentina and they were in France'.*

In Sarah's case it took her German long-term boyfriend to make her start reading in German. Her love for reading developed when she started being educated in English, and most of the books she has read are in English. She finds reading in German much more challenging and culturally different. More recently, however, during a long-term relationship with a German boyfriend, she not only read more in German but even got into German poetry during this relationship (Goethe) and she read some parts of Faust, and enjoyed listening to her partner reading it in German. She tried to read some parts of Faust in English, but it did not feel the same.

Marion today reads Welsh on the internet and when she is in Wales she buys women's magazines in Welsh. She also writes emails in Welsh to her cousins in Canada. *'Email has been a great benefit and I think nobody cares how you write, you can put English words in if you don't know a Welsh one'.*

Ingrid overcame her feeling that she had missed out on some aspects of Swedish culture due to her (Swedish) father's death when she was 11, and Ingrid does read Swedish books, listens to Swedish music, and watches Swedish films as much as she reads American or British literature and so on.

Similarly, Saad watches Kurdish and Arabic TV and films and listens to both Kurdish and Arabic music, and Fatima watches Arabic TV to keep up with what is happening back home and also to show her children the way that Eid celebrations are different in Morocco. She also watches soap operas in Arabic from time to time, and enjoys listening to Moroccan music.

Sophie said: *'I have a Google home page in every language; French, English, Spanish, and Italian and I constantly switch between the languages, (except Occitan because there's no one for me to speak it with,) that's the frame of mind I'm in'.*

In contrast, Mohammed feels that his upbringing focused on language, but didn't include wider culture: *'I would have hoped that I could have kept up my Bengali and Arabic in a way that would have meant that I could read in Bengali and Arabic for pleasure. I wish I had an appreciation of those languages – from novels to music to art – I didn't get access to the whole culture – it was more about formal learning and gave me a top-heavy view of the language. I think that my parents could have done more to cultivate a love of those languages, rather than feeling that learning the language was a necessity'.*

Christine (whose German mother stopped speaking German to her in France when she was about six) also similarly regrets that she rarely watches a German film or reads a book in German, and now feels that if her mother had pursued speaking German with her, she would be more likely to access German culture and her German heritage.

Tom had more or less given up reading any Croatian when he moved to Australia, and this lasted for around 25 years, but he did restart later in life. This occurred when war broke out in what was then Yugoslavia, including Croatia. Tom started buying papers in Croatian to follow what was happening. Since then, the development of the internet has also helped him to have access to reading material in Croatian: *'It felt good, even though I found that the language changed so much in that time from when I stopped reading'.*

Conclusion

Most interviewees did still access the culture of both of their languages. Those that did not almost always regretted this. Reading fictional books in a language for pleasure was the most important cultural activity mentioned, followed by films and then music. This again underlines the importance of ensuring that children learnt to read and write in both/all of their languages. It is also clear that the ability to read and write is different from the willingness to read in a language for pleasure. Some interviewees who could read still did not feel able to do so, perhaps because it was more difficult for them than reading in another stronger language.

27 Accents

When the team started out on this project, I, at least, certainly assumed that interviewees who had learnt several languages from a young age would not have an accent in either or any of their languages. This is one reason cited in some books about bilingualism as to why parents should be consistent and start from birth, and not wait and start speaking a language when the child is a bit older.

Most of our interviewees did end up speaking both or all of their languages without any distinctive foreign accent, but there were four clear exceptions among the interviewees who did have clearly identifiable accents in one or other language. Quite a large group of interviewees said that although they did not have a foreign accent per se, they sounded somehow international, posh or different from many native speakers. Some said this might be because they did not have a local or regional accent that most native speakers would have. Some, although they had no accent, were still clearly identifiable as having learned a language abroad when they returned home on visits. This was because their language input had been isolated and they had not kept up with the ways that the language had changed in the home country in their absence. They often sounded a bit dated, did not use the latest slang or sounded too formal or correct in their language use.

Some interviewees revelled in the fact that they spoke a language without an accent. Saadia, for instance, who only started speaking Urdu when she was around 11, commented: '...when I spoke Urdu, I used to love the fact that people couldn't tell that I was born here [the UK] – I speak as if I could have been brought up in India. I was sometimes asked where I am from or how much I have studied in Urdu. . . . I can make out that I am not from here [laughs]'.

Similarly, Ingrid said: '. . . I do feel privileged that I can slip in and out of two societies. I have never had anyone in the States ask me if I was foreign, nor in Sweden'.

Many other interviewees who did not have accents just took this for granted. Like monolinguals, many of our interviewees had several accents which they used at different times; you may remember Mohammed learning to speak cockney English as a child to fit in at school, as well as the more formal English that his father spoke sometimes at home (see p.90). Similarly, Marion speaks Welsh without an accent and has two accents in English: 'I'm talking to you in my "work" accent, but I think when I go to Wales I change and I talk English like that [with a Welsh accent]'.

Another issue that arose during our interviews is the form of language the interviewees used to compare their speech to, in order to decide if they have a noticeable accent. Pedro would not have any noticeable accent in Texas where he grew up, but he says an American audience listening to him speak in English could tell that he is also a Hispanic speaker because of his way of speaking. Certainly to an audience in England he has only an American accent when he speaks English. In Spain, people sometimes think that he is from Latin America, perhaps Colombia, when he speaks Spanish.

Similarly, Bindi, who remembers losing her accent and adopting London English when her family moved to England when she was around 11, would not stand out amongst Gujarati speakers from Kenya, but she says that she has an East African accent that is noticeable to Gujarati speakers from India.

Five interviewees said that they sounded international in some way in one of their languages. So Susanne, for example, said: *As to accent, people can't place me. They can't tell I'm not German, but they can tell the intonation is not quite right for somebody who is from Germany'.* Camilla said she feels that she has a slight accent, although people she speaks to in Danish do not know that she is not a native Danish speaker (if she sounds a little odd, friends have told her that Danish people might wonder what mix of regional Danish accents she has).

Kwesi said that the English they were taught in Ghana was the Queen's English, in that it was very structured, very formal and proper. He noticed when he moved to England that the language had moved on. When he worked during holidays at hotels or food shops, people would say, *'God you sound so posh!'* On the other hand, Kwesi had the same problem when in Ghana where they seemed to think that he had an accent, and assumed that he had been raised abroad. (He was, in fact brought up in Ghana, but at a private school where he mixed with lots of children of expatriates working in Ghana that were originally from elsewhere.)

Interviewees who said that their language sounded somehow out of date included Vera W (speaking Chinese) who said that the Cantonese speakers she meets notice that she speaks in an old-fashioned or quaint way. She probably speaks the language as it was spoken a few decades ago when her parents left China, and the language has since moved on. This may have been accentuated by the fact that the family was unable to visit China for many years. Mohammed also did not travel back to Bangladesh during his childhood: *'When I went to Bangladesh, [for the first time when he was 18] even though I speak Sylheti very well, people could tell I was from London – even though I don't have an accent'.* Mohammed explains that the versions of language spoken here and in Bangladesh have changed so that there are now subtle differences in usage and vocabulary, so that people from London are easily identified by their different phrases and usage. Antony also felt that his Greek was slightly old-fashioned.

Armelle actually told us that she had sometimes wished that she did have an accent, as this would prevent disputes about her identity with people she meets. She speaks both French and Spanish without any foreign accent. As her mother is from Argentina, she speaks Spanish with an Argentinean accent. Armelle feels that she is French. When she tells people in Argentina that she is French, they often do not believe her because she does not have a French accent when speaking Spanish. Armelle finds this common denial of her actual identity to be difficult and upsetting, and sometimes wishes she had a tiny French accent in Spanish to avoid this problem.

Those adults who do have an accent are more likely to have been those that had less input in a language as children (but some of the children who had very little input also ended up without accents, and some of the children with considerable input ended up *with* accents). In some cases, the interviewees may not have had any native speaker models without a foreign accent to listen to and imitate. So Emilio says he has a slight accent in English and no accent in Spanish. Emilio grew up in Argentina and learnt his Spanish through a bilingual school there. He mentioned that all of the teachers could also speak Spanish, and they may well have spoken English with Spanish accents. Similarly, Adeyinka, who learnt his English at school in Nigeria, was taught for the most part by Nigerians (he remembers only one teacher from the United States at one point). He has a slight accent when he speaks English.

Sophie, who grew up in south-west France hearing, but hardly speaking, the very marginalised Occitan language, says that she has a French accent in Occitan but no accent when she speaks French. Charles, whose mother stopped speaking Dutch to him when he was quite small (he does not remember exactly when), says that he has a French accent when he speaks Dutch. Astrid, who learnt German entirely through a six-month visit to Germany and three or four years of a German Saturday school, says: *'Some people say I sound American, some people say they know I am not German. . .a lot of people say my accent is quite good'.*

Tom and Sabina are exceptions; although Tom heard exclusively Croatian until he was 11, he says that he now has a slight English accent when he speaks Croatian, while Sabina had heard and spoken Urdu at home until her mother died when she was nine, and she started responding to her father in English. Two years later her father remarried a monolingual Urdu speaker, and Sabina had to relearn speaking Urdu. Although she speaks Urdu fluently now, she does say that she has a definite accent and *'people in Pakistan always know that I am from abroad as soon as I speak'.*

Vera C began life speaking mainly English while living with her parents in France and being looked after by her English grandmother. She lived in France until her late teens, attending both English and French schools at different times. She fled France in 1939 when she was 19 and applied to join the air force as a volunteer to help the war effort and was told: *'. . . don't go anywhere [in England] where you have to talk because no on will understand you'.* She says, *'Evidently, I had an awful accent!'* She also told us that when she later married and first visited her husband's relatives in Yorkshire, she could not understand them and neither could they understand her. And she heard that they referred to her as *'a foreigner'.*

Helen was the only child who said that she had an accent in both of her languages. She grew up in Holland with her Dutch mother and English father and preferred to speak only Dutch except during visits to her relatives in England (who did not speak Dutch). Helen has a Dutch accent when she speaks English, but she also says that people say that she has a slight accent when she speaks Dutch.

Conclusion

Just as some children are gifted mimics, some children will find it easier to imitate speech exactly and without any accent. It does seem as though children who are raised with interrupted input or lower levels of input in a language are somewhat more likely to end up with an accent. (Thus Sophie's Occitan is accented, and Sabina's Urdu has an accent.) In all but one case, though, the child only had an accent in the weaker of their two languages. And having said that, several of the children that had very limited input (e.g. Christine) did not have any accent at all. As mentioned above, speaking without an accent is sometimes linked to the age that a child starts learning a language. Our group does not support this, as none of the children who migrated later (Tom, 11, Fatima, 10 and Mumtaz, 7) speaks the language that they learnt after they moved (all English) with an accent, whereas two of the children who learnt languages from birth, and one who learnt it aged three or four do, as adults, have slight accents. There was also no clear link between visiting a country regularly and not having an accent. Similarly, of the children who resisted speaking a language to their parents, four do not have accents, and only one does. In our experience, many parents feel that the priority is that a child can speak without grammatical errors, with some fluency, that they can read and write to some extent, and a perfect accent is probably a lower priority. In any event, it is very unclear what a parent can actually do if a child does speak with a noticeable accent.

- The only tip that we can pass on is that your child(ren) may speak with a noticeably dated form of the language if they do not visit a country regularly and/or meet recent migrants or visitors from that country.

28 Learning Additional Languages

When we designed our original base questionnaire (see Annex 1, p.232), we forgot to include a question about whether our interviewees had noticed any impact of their bilingualism on learning additional foreign languages. Despite this, many interviewees spontaneously mentioned this issue – and so we did then start to ask our last interviewees about this. About a third of interviewees mentioned this. The large majority were entirely positive, while two were in some way a mixture of positive and negative. There is some evidence from the academic community that children who are already bilingual may be able to learn an additional language more easily. There are a variety of theories as to why this might be the case – ranging from changes in brain development due to hearing two languages, to the idea that these children just have a great deal of confidence in their ability to learn languages. The examples in our group included relatively straightforward examples of benefits from pronunciation, or in terms of vocabulary with shared roots, but also included benefits from interviewees who had learnt languages that are completely unrelated.

I will start with the more straightforward examples. Saad spoke Kurdish at home and Arabic in the community and at school. He learnt English as a foreign language at school. Saad was aware that he was better than many of the other (monolingual Arabic-speaking) students in his class at English. He noticed that bilingual students had a less strong accent when speaking English. Also, Arabic does not contain the sound 'p', whereas Kurdish does. Arabic speakers have a lot of difficulty separating 'b' and 'p' in English, whereas Kurdish speakers do not have this problem.

Benefits from shared roots, giving advantages in terms of vocabulary or grammar, were also common. So Sophie felt that her knowledge of Occitan helped her to learn Spanish and Italian, and when Snjezana started in her Italian-medium school in Croatia with no prior knowledge of Italian and no transitional help, she learnt Italian very quickly at school and feels that the fact that she could already speak Esperanto helped her in this. In Charles's case, he used his childhood languages to help him learn other foreign languages: 'With French it was easy to learn Italian later on in life. With Dutch it was easier to learn German, Luxembourgian and English. I understand Spanish and I understand some Portuguese as well. . . . I think having bilingual education made it easier to learn different languages and also made it easier to operate in international environments'.

An example that specifically referred to grammar is that that of (Greek and English bilingual) Antony, who learned some French and a little bit of German at secondary school. He felt he was not the brightest in the class but he wished he had continued. He believes that being bilingual helped him to learn additional languages; for instance, he tried to apply the masculine gender Greek logic to the French language and, although it did not work, he feels that being bilingual gave him more resources in terms of manipulating language. Antony's knowledge of Greek and its masculine/feminine distinction would have given Antony an advantage over monolingual English children who had no knowledge of any such system (even if the logic that applied in Greek in operating the system could not be transferred to French).

Examples which are of more interest to linguists because it is much harder to understand how they come about are those where, even if languages are completely unrelated, with no shared vocabulary or grammar, children who are already bilingual seem to find it easier to learn a third language. So, for example, Sylvia said she does think that being bilingual has probably helped her to learn other languages as an adult. She has been able to quickly learn enough to get by in many other European languages, which she partly puts down to being able to use the common roots of many words and similar grammar systems, but she also agrees that this was also the case with a language like Turkish (which does not share either vocabulary or grammatical systems with the languages that Syliva is bilingual in – English and French). Here she says that even then her knowledge and understanding of the systems that underpin language may well have helped her.

Bindi herself did not remember that being bilingual helped her learn French or Latin at school, but today, 'As a parent I can see how my children [bilingual in English and Gujarati] are able to switch . . . they are much more flexible in their thinking and both my children are doing very well in French'.

Markus felt that: 'I think that being bilingual helps you to learn languages. On a simple level you understand that things are said differently in different languages and you understand that different languages work differently. So switching between languages is constant and so the mental approach to learning a language is easier. So when you are bilingual you are more aware of the different structures and you think about language more, and you are used to the idea of having different languages in your head, in a way, which I think are the advantages'.

Other interviewees simply report that they were able to pick up language very easily, so Vera W had private French lessons with a local teacher (whilst still of primary school age) and she reached a very high-level for her age with relative ease. She now regrets that she did not keep this up – the lessons were dropped when the family moved. Pedro's impressive language learning occurred as an adult when he joined the US military, which sent him to Korea and Germany where he learned to speak both languages very well.

Two interviewees mentioned that although being bilingual was partially beneficial, it may also have had a downside; in both cases this concerned the fact that, as both interviewees were used to speaking several languages to a very high standard, they were somewhat perfectionist. Ingrid was the daughter of a Swedish father and American mother who spent the first two years of her life in Mexico where she learnt to speak Spanish (which was in fact the only language she would actively speak as a very young child). The family moved to live in Sweden and Ingrid forgot her Spanish. Nonetheless, when Ingrid started to learn Spanish much later as a foreign language, she does feel that, in some ways, and although she did not remember anything from her early childhood, it seemed relatively easy to cope with the different word order and that she was able to speak it with a minimal accent. She lived in Spain for six months as an adult and was quite comfortable speaking Spanish by the end of this time. She did say though that the fact that she spoke two languages fluently may have inhibited her Spanish: 'I think also since I have both English and Swedish, I would be so self-conscious that it should be perfect that it would take me forever just to say something'.

We mentioned earlier that, in Snjezana's case, she attributes the perfectionism that she has about speaking languages that she is not totally comfortable in to the style of teaching that was used at her school. Snjezana feels that the school's ethos did not encourage creativity or exploration, and children were expected to be passive learners. Combined with this, Snjezana feels sensitive about making mistakes when she speaks in a language she does not speak fluently – and she attributes this to be being corrected and reprimanded a lot at school: 'I learnt German as well at school and at the point when I stopped learning it I had a very solid high or intermediate level. However I stopped using it. . . . I will choose the language based on the ones I speak best, rather than what is best suited to the occasion'.

Conclusion

Overall our sample agreed that bilinguals may find it easier to learn additional languages. Our interviewees suggested a wide range of factors that may be involved. Clearly if children are learning a language that is related to a language that they already speak, they may benefit from shared grammar, shared vocabulary or shared writing systems. But parents can take heart from the fact that, even if the child is learning a language that is completely unrelated to any language that they already speak, a child who is already bilingual may find this easier than a monolingual child. This may be because bilingual children are simply more aware of language, and take it less for granted, or it may be because their brains are wired slightly differently, or it may just be because they are less intimidated and more confident about their ability to learn languages. There is some evidence from within our interviews that supports this view.

PART 6

Overall Analysis and Recommendations

29 Factors Linked to Success or Failure

When I first started to think about the contents of this chapter, I was quite frustrated as there seem to be no simple correlations. Even factors that one would think were quite straightforward turn out to be more complex. So, take, for example, the interviewees who stopped getting any significant input in a language after a certain point – some retained their languages, and some did not. Even if there might seem to be a pattern in terms of one factor, there will still be one or more exceptions that indicate that this is not decisive. Although somewhat frustrating for me in writing this chapter, looking at it from the other end, this indicates that almost any barrier, problem or difficulty can be overcome, which is, in fact, quite inspiring for parents. We know anecdotally from our work in the Waltham Forest Bilingual Group and in the community that there are two main reasons why children who could potentially have been bilingual end up monolingual: the first is that their parents decided not to speak the minority language to them, and the second is that the parents started to speak a language but decided to give up because there were setbacks or they got bad advice. It is therefore quite helpful for parents who do embark on this project to know that other children have overcome problems, that low points do pass, and that it was not all plain sailing for other families.

That said, I would not take the fact that Christine learnt German even though her mother stopped speaking it to her aged six as a model to emulate. Such exceptions may have been interviewees who were very talented in terms of learning languages, and it may well be that a child with different aptitudes would have struggled in the same situation.

One interviewee also pointed out (I suspect correctly) that a child's personality may affect the results: *'I was excruciatingly shy at school. And I think that if I had been a different child, I would probably speak a lot more Danish now. I think it comes from me being shy. My sister had less Danish input than me, but she is much more extrovert and confident, and she is really confident speaking Danish. With my Danish, really it's a lack of confidence . . . I can speak it if I'm pushed. I think a more confident child who had my bilingual childhood, may well have ended up speaking a lot more Danish than I do'.*

There are a great many variables and our sample is far too small to draw very many definitive conclusions.

I am not going to exhaustively point out every single factor that does not seem to correlate with any final outcome whether positive or negative. But I will go through the factors that, from my experience in helping to run a group supporting parents in bilingual families, are ones that parents often worry about.

Factors That Do Not Seem to Be Decisive

(1) If your child(ren) prefer not to speak one of their languages to you, this does not mean all is lost. Interviewees who resisted speaking one or both parents' preferred languages all ended up fluent speakers of that language (in one case less confidently). (See p.81 onwards.) In all of these cases, at least one parent was a first language speaker of the language, and continued to speak it to the child. In all cases, although the children's responses in another language were acceptable to the parent, the child still knew that the parent would have preferred that the response was in another language. Another group of interviewees were in a slightly different situation whereby they never spoke one language (or not after a certain age) but this was totally accepted by their parents to the extent that the interviewees were not aware that the parent had a preference. These interviewees in our sample did not always end up speaking as fluently.

(2) There was no difference in mixed-language families between families where the father spoke the minority language and families where the mother spoke the minority language. In both cases, interviewees grew up speaking the minority language fluently (see p.16).

(3) Most interviewees hearing/speaking marginalised/perceived low status languages still retained that language (e.g. Saad, Marion, Josune). Sophie's experience of speaking Occitan is the exception (for more on her story, see p.149).

(4) Interviewees who did not learn to read and write in one of their languages as children did still acquire a good verbal knowledge – many opted to learn to read and write as adults. All but one interviewee regretted later, once adult, not having learnt to read and write as children (see p.134). Interviewees whilst children would all have preferred to not attend Saturday language schools. However, interviewees who dropped out of such schools universally regretted this as adults. Interviewees who did continue in Saturday language schools were glad that they had – once they were adults.

(5) It was surprising to me how many interviewees were able to function very comfortably in a language as adults despite having quite limited input either in totality or after a certain point (see, for example, Christine p.57, Daniela p.50 & 163).

(6) Interviewees whose parents raised them with a strict language division were successful; only one interviewee described resenting this as a child, although this did not prevent her going to some lengths to speak the same minority language to her children. Equally successful were interviewees who had some rules but these were more relaxed.

(7) Interviewees whose parents switched the language they spoke to them midway through their childhoods were also successful. In some cases, this was to rebalance the language input that interviewees had after a move between countries, so Markus's family spoke mostly German at home whilst living in the United States, but more English at home whilst living in Germany. However, in some cases

where a parent gave up speaking a language and the child had limited or no other input in that language, it was partially or totally lost (e.g. Daniela and Italian; Aimee and Mina).

(8)   Provided that they started school at preschool or reception/first grade, interviewees who entered the education system not able to understand or speak the language used at school did not remember any sustained disadvantage or problems. There were certainly no long-term educational disadvantages for these interviewees. Many were subsequently very high academic achievers – Sylvia went to Oxford University, several have PhDs. One child who understood English but preferred to speak Welsh when she started school (Marion) did feel that her early years of schooling were adversely affected. The problems were resolved when the family moved to Wales and she moved to a school where the teachers spoke Welsh as well as English. It is unclear what might have been the outcome if she had stayed in London.

(9)   Our sample included interviewees with highly educated parents as well as those with parents who were literate but who had not completed school up to age 16, as well as some whose parents were not literate in any language. All groups successfully raised multilingual children.

Factors Where There is a Mixed Picture

(10)   Interviewees whose parents freely mixed languages were also successful. In many cases, these interviewees also functioned in environments outside the home in both languages where mixing was not acceptable (e.g. Markus mixed German and English at home but at different times attended both English and German medium-schools where mixing was not acceptable). Parvati very usefully described how having monolingual Hindi-speaking carers and visitors forced her to stop inserting the odd English word into Hindi sentences and helped her to raise her Hindi to a new level. We only had one example of a child growing up with quite a lot of mixing at home where, in the case of one of his languages, there was not an environment where he needed to speak that language without mixing. Pedro, who grew up in a bilingual Spanish/English community, had to learn to speak English at school without mixing, but (despite the efforts of his father) was more used to mixing English and Spanish languages at home – there was not an equivalent place where if he mixed an English word into a Spanish sentence this would be unacceptable or he would not be understood. When Pedro lived in Spain as an adult, he noticed that he would often want to use one English word in an otherwise fluent Spanish sentence. Pedro would recommend that parents should not mix languages if possible, saying that it is easy to mix them if you speak separate languages, whereas it can be hard to separate them if you are used to mixing them a lot of the time.

(11)   Interviewees who moved into an educational system using a language medium that they had no understanding of after the age of seven were more likely to have

had problems. Daniela overcame these quickly in her French-language boarding school, as did Shadi in Sweden. Tom, who arrived in Australia aged 12 speaking only Croatian overcame these, but he had to work very hard to do so. Fatima (moved age 10 and missed one year of school entirely) and Mumtaz (moved aged seven, but faced significant additional difficulties linked to her mother's ill health) did not totally overcome the problems – both learnt very fluent English, but both felt that they did less well in exams than they might otherwise have done.

(12)   None of our interviewees reported any problem learning the majority language fluently, except where the majority language was not also the school language (e.g. Charles who learnt Luxembourgian from the community ended up with a limited knowledge of the language). Velji learnt Swahili from the streets, but in his case this was supplemented as he used it during many years for his work, while Armelle learnt Italian from the community, her friends and the TV. We have heard of other examples whereby children have not learnt a majority language where it is not also the medium of education (e.g. a child in a well-off family in Pakistan educated at an English-medium school, and where the parents spoke in English who reached adulthood with a limited knowledge of Urdu).

(13)   We were also struck by the complexity of the interviewees' responses to questions about their identities, and their feelings of belonging or not. Not everyone reported any issue here, but quite a high number did. If we try to isolate one factor that links all those that did or which distinguishes between the group that did and the group that did not, again we cannot find any particular link or factor. Several interviewees used the term 'rootless', or referred to having moved several times. However, Claudia moved the most times between the most places as a child but still had one of the firmest identities. Some of the interviewees who reported feeling 'rootless' had not actually moved themselves, but had felt that their parents belonged somewhere that they did not live. Both children of migrants and mixed-language families reported issues around identity.

(14)   Examples where interviewees did partially or totally lose (third) languages resulted from their parents deciding to stop speaking to them in that language (but in some cases the interviewees still did not lose the language) and/or separation from parents or a change in circumstance that meant that they had no continuing exposure to that language for some years (again, some still interviewees retained languages when this happened), and one instance where a adult can understand but not speak a highly marginalised language.

30 Recommendations to Parents Raising Multilingual Children

Hundreds of questions and issues arise in this subject area and for a comprehensive and textbook answer to every question we would suggest that you buy or borrow Colin Baker's *A Parents' and Teachers' Guide to Bilingualism* (see 'Further Reading'). Here we take just 11 key areas (A to K), each of which is a subject that comes up very often and on which our findings shed some light. We give details of some recommendations on and around each key area.

I will make four important points first:

(1) As stated in the introduction to this book: there are no 'off the shelf' solutions. Every family is different. (In fact every child is different.) You need to think through all the different aspects of your particular situation, the resources that you have available to you, and your family's particular constraints. You need to work out what feels comfortable for you, what you can sustain, and what you can do and still feel true to yourself.

(2) Given sufficient motivation yourself, children who have at least an average ability to learn languages and who you can motivate, you can break any rule, ignore any piece of advice and still succeed. For example, a child who finds it relatively easy to mimic people or who practises enough to do so well, will generally be able to speak without an accent even if the input they have had has been lower than the ideal level. Many of our interviewees' families did not follow one or many of the pieces of advice that follow but still had successful outcomes. The less you are motivated, and the less you are able to motivate your children, the higher *the risk* that, if you break rules, this will have an impact on the relative strength of the languages your child speaks or even if they continue to speak both or all of the languages at all.

(3) Some of these recommendations relate straightforwardly to the findings of our interviews. However, some sections also involve me using judgements relying on the hundreds of conversations I have had with parents and children at our group's drop-in sessions and other events. (So although several of our interviewees were successfully raised as bilinguals with very limited input in one language, we are not recommending this because our experience and conversations suggest that it would not be at all wise to rely on this as a general rule!)

(4) If your child has a significant physical or learning disability or behaviour issues, some of this advice may not be appropriate and you should really seek individual guidance from a qualified source. We would suggest that a speech therapist who has specialised in bilingual issues would be a good first step.

(A.) Deciding which languages to speak to your child(ren) from before they are born/whilst they are under three months old. (If your children are already over three months see Section C 'Changing the language you speak to your child')

(A 1) Think carefully about which language(s) you are going to use to talk to your child (if possible, in advance). If you speak only one language well, confidently and fluently, then you should speak that language to your child. However, some of you may have a choice. You need to be sure that you can speak any language that you plan to speak to your children very well, but this does not mean that it necessarily *has* to be a language that you spoke or heard yourself as a child – as several of our interviewees demonstrated. (See Claudia whose German mother decided to speak English to her, p. 21). Bear in mind that although your conversations may initially seem fairly basic (but including songs, nursery rhymes or poems if at all possible), children do need rich and fluent language input, and the complexity and range of the language, and the concepts and subtleties you will need will increase as your children get older. With toddlers you will need to be able to respond *instantaneously* in this language and be very clear (e.g. when your child is about to run into a road or has just somehow reached up and grabbed a sharp knife). Later on, you may need to discuss quite sophisticated topics with them and you will need to hold your own in heated discussions – but don't worry about vocabulary too much. Many of us learn for the first time or need reminding of a lot of vocabulary from our children. When your children are around five you may find yourself learning names of dinosaurs (e.g. Plesiosaur), or geological eras (e.g. Triassic). When your children are aged around nine, you might find yourself discussing Quidditch, or equivalent fractions. And so it goes on...

Once you have decided which language to speak you can guess or estimate the input your child will get from different languages and see how balanced this will be. Parents often think mainly in terms of the input from parents and carers, whereas in reality, even from a very young age, children are absorbing information from the whole world around them. (So Ingrid, who was raised until she was two in Mexico listening to her parents speaking to her in English and Swedish, still preferred to only speak Spanish which she heard at a nursery and in the community.) Your child will get input from each adult he or she spends time with, siblings, other relatives (e.g. grandparents or cousins or close family friends), the community, and later on, mainstream schools, any additional schools as well as holidays. You can just write a simple list. Or you can go further and estimate how much time the child will spend hearing or speaking each language from all of these sources (see examples on pages 212 & 213). Here we have put up to five ticks for each item on the list, loosely based on the amount of time the child spends doing it, whether it involves a lot of talking and listening, and how important it is to the child him or herself. (Clearly these are just guesses; this is just to give you some idea). A blank table is included in Annex 3.

If you do this before your child is born it would be worth checking it a few months later to see how things have turned out in reality. Likewise, if there are other significant changes, you can update it.

Although the impact of factors outside the home (school, community) will be more limited when your child is young, you need to also think about the situation when your child is a little older as you will probably not want to change the language that you speak. In the examples in Figures 30.1 and 30.2 (pages 212 and 213), we have estimated the input when the child is two and again when the child is eight. We do appreciate that many people cannot see ahead for eight years or more and predict all these circumstances, but we think it is better to try this than to just let things happen.

The last row of the table allows you to allocate some points linked to the strength of your child's emotions about people who speak that language or its culture or heroes. This could be people s/he is particularly close to, or things he or she particularly admires. So the fact that a sports hero speaks Urdu or the fact that a favourite song is sung in Hindi or Spanish might be significant to your child.

Ideally this will give you an overview of whether input in each language will be reasonably balanced. If you can achieve a ratio that is within the range of 60:40 (without fixing the scores) then you can relax (for now) and be very grateful. (You can only relax 'for now' because there is no magic number whereby if your balance is more even than 60:40 you are guaranteed a good outcome – your child may be particularly shy or want desperately to fit in, or your situation may change etc.) An imbalance in favour of the minority language (i.e. the language not normally spoken in the community which is more usual in the early years before school starts) is less of a problem than an imbalance in favour of the majority language, as the impact of the community in many societies can be very strong, even overwhelming. (However, if your majority language is perceived as lower status and is not the language used in schools, this would be more worrying – this could arise somewhere like India, where the school language may be English, with the majority language Hindi or a regional language. In these circumstances the majority language might well be more vulnerable.)

If your ratio is more like 75% in one language and 25% in the other, then you can either try to make some changes by adding in time spent with people speaking the language that has scored lowest (see A 2 and A 3 below). If this is difficult, you can look at somehow making sure that whoever is providing the child's 25% input ensures that this time is very rich in terms of language input. The amount and richness of language interaction is probably more important than the crude amount of time – so if one parent sees the child for less time, but still spends much of the time they do have together talking, listening or reading with the child, actively playing games involving language, singing nursery rhymes and other high-quality language interactions, this can also help to ensure a high-level of input.

It is important to note that although we talk here in terms of balance, this is not a zero-sum situation (i.e. it is not a competition between the languages). A very full and rich input in one language does not prevent a child learning a second language (in fact the opposite is almost certainly true), so as a parent you need never and should never deliberately reduce the richness or amount of language a child gets in any language.

If your input in each language is likely to be even less balanced than a ratio of 75:25, you need to acknowledge that there is a risk that your child will be much stronger in one language than the other. This is a risk in that it may happen for some children,

Child aged two	Language A	Language B	Language C	
	Urdu	English	none	
Loosely based on the number of hours the child spends				
With mother	√√√√			Mother does not work and spends most time with the child
With father	√√			Father home mainly evenings and weekends
With childminder				
Interacting with siblings	√√	√√		Elder brother home after school and weekends, speaks mixture of English and Urdu
Preschool group		√		Once a week
Time spent with relatives	√√			At least one day a week spent with grandparents
Other forms of input				
Regular holidays in Urdu environment				Not possible at this time
Community		√√		Although not a huge amount of time, still given quite a lot of significance
Language father uses to mother	√			
Language mother uses to father	√			
Particular relationships/positive emotions	√√√√			
	18	6		75% Urdu to 25% English

Figure 30.1 Example of an estimate of a child's input in different languages at the age of two

Child aged eight	Language A	Language B	Language C	
	Urdu	English	none	
Loosely based on the number of hours the child spends				
With mother	√√			Now reduced as mother is now working and child is at school
With father	√√			
School		√√√√√		30+ hours per week in school
With childminder		√√		Two nights after school per week
Interacting with siblings	√	√√		Brother is now keener to speak English than Urdu
Time spent with relatives	√			
Other (swimming, kung fu, drama)		√√√		
Regular holidays in Urdu environment	√√√			
Community		√√√		
Language father uses to mother	√			
Language mother uses to father	√			
Particular relationships/positive emotions	√√√	√√		The child now has close emotional ties with school friends as well as with his or her immediate family
Total	14	17		45% Urdu to 55% English

Figure 30.2 Example of an estimate of a child's input in different languages at the age of eight

while for others it will not; however, it will be more likely to happen in this situation than if the child had more input in the second language. But as children get older and as your circumstances change there may still be ways in which you can support and boost a weaker language. We saw this with interviewees who went to school in a minority language, with Parvati to some extent in her teens, and with the children of migrants who moved aged 7, 10 and 12 and still acquired a fluent language from a zero start after those ages. In some of our families with successful outcomes, the input that the child received was always limited to one parent, and if we had estimated input for some of them they could have been well under 25% input from one language. So it can be done. If you are raising your children trilingually, then you can still do this exercise and see how the balance between the languages is likely to work. Again if any one language goes below 25%, you may want to try to adjust things or ensure that this time is spent doing a lot of talking and listening with your child.

(A 2) If your child is less than three months old, and you can easily change things so that the input in different languages is more even, then do so. If your child is over three months old, see recommendation C.

(A 3) Do not assume you will easily speak the language that you choose if you are not using it regularly already – particularly if it is one of several languages that you speak – try to get some practice in before your child is born. Try to get back into the habit of speaking that language regularly. If you do not have anyone to speak it to (and do not fancy talking to yourself!), you could try immersing yourself in that culture through films, books, music and the internet for a few months leading up to your child's birth.

(A 4) If one parent is going to speak to the child(ren) in a language that the other does not understand, think about whether the second parent might be able to start to learn that language. You do not need to be able to read or write in it. You do not even necessarily need to be able to speak it. If you can gather sufficient knowledge to understand a simple conversation, this will really help later on. (It will mean that when your spouse or partner says 'No you can't have a biscuit right now because you didn't eat all your lunch but you can have an apple if you are hungry', and the child comes to you minutes later and asks the same question, you will be able to give the same answer.) Learning at least a passive knowledge of a language alongside babies and children is not a pipe dream. We know several people in our group and beyond who have actually achieved this – and not only understand but actively now speak an additional language. In our sample, Josune reports learning some Czech solely from the language between her husband and her children, but you may well want to do more than this and actively study it – you may have time for an evening class or the money for a language course on CD or tape, and if you have neither, your spouse or partner could always start to teach you (in which case he or she can focus particularly on the vocabulary used to, and about, babies and young children). Once you start hearing your spouse talk to your child, this will reinforce what you have already learnt and, as you hear words you do not know, you can note them and ask for translations. The vocabulary used to talk to babies and very small children is usually quite limited and it may well be quite easy to learn to understand and say, with a minimum amount of work on your part to keep up with your child – particularly if your aim is mainly to be able to understand conversations.

(A 5) If the fact that you are speaking to your child in a language which your parents did not speak to you worries you at all, try to put this worry aside. Many parents in our sample of interviewees successfully and happily raised children whilst speaking to them in a language which their parents never spoke to them. (However, if you do not know children's rhymes, songs and lullabies and so on you may want to try to get hold of and learn some of those – many parents re-learn nursery rhymes that they may have learnt themselves as toddlers but have since forgotten. New rhymes are also added all the time, so the fact that you did not know them as a child is absolutely no barrier if you make the effort to learn them.) Some people said to us, though, that they had tried speaking to their children in a language that their parents had not spoken to them when they were children but that it just felt too unnatural, so you might feel this, at least at the beginning.

(A 6) Whatever language pattern you have decided to use, start from day one – the longer you leave it the harder it will be to switch.

(A 7) Use terms for parents, grandparents, aunts, and uncles from the language that those relatives speak (assuming that this is one of the languages your children speak). For example, in a family where the mother speaks English and the father French, the mother might say 'That's papa's shirt', and not 'That's daddy's shirt'.

(A 8) If you are raising children with a spouse or a partner, make a conscious decision about how to raise your children bilingually and agree on it. Do not allow language to be an area of dispute between parents. Talk about it, but particularly if you do not totally agree all the time, do it out of the hearing of the children. Marion was deeply affected by what she saw as a language rift within her family. If one parent is mildly snobbish towards or disparages the language that another parent is speaking to their child, the child will almost certainly notice and make a note, and a number of our interviewees remembered this (e.g. Marion and Parvati).

(A 9) Again, if you are part of a couple, it can be very useful to ask yourselves and agree between you *why* you want your children to be bilingual. Some parents really just want their children to be able to communicate with relatives (e.g. Josune wants her children to speak Basque so as to be part of her extended Basque family. Reading and writing is less important). For these parents, the primary focus may be on understanding and participating in ordinary family activities. However, others know that their stay in a country is time limited and plan to move elsewhere where the children will need to be able to attend school in another language. Here the parents probably want the child to be able to read and write as well as speak fluently about the range of topics that might come up at school. If you know *why* you want your children to be bilingual, this will help you to make lots of difficult decisions later on. You can then prioritise both between different ways of using language and, when time pressures become significant as children get older, between an additional language and other activities. If your child has one weaker language that they use less often, would you prefer that they had the vocabulary for games to play with their cousins or the vocabulary to function in school? Should they have seen the latest Bollywood film or be able to write an essay? Later on, should they give up a language Saturday school so as to be able to train in a sport where they show promise or to spend time practising a musical instrument?

(B) Changing the language that you speak between yourselves:

(B 1) Another way of adjusting the input that your children receive in different languages is to adjust the languages the adults around the child speak to each other. If you can comfortably do so, then it is useful if the adults around the child can speak to each other in the language that the child will otherwise get less input in, which is normally the language that is not spoken in the community. (Bindi and her husband deliberately switched from speaking English to speaking Gujarati to each other in front of their children.) If you are going to try to change this, be aware that for some people it is really difficult to break a long-established habit (others find it less difficult). Trying to make this change when you have just had your first child, and may not be getting a full night's sleep and are adjusting to a major life change, may not be the wisest course if you have a choice! So again, this is a good reason to discuss this in the first or second trimesters of pregnancy, and try to start making the changes then.

(B 2) Do not assume that both parents have to listen and answer in the same language. If both parents understand both languages but they cannot comfortably carry on a conversation in the language that you would prefer, it is possible for one parent to speak always in one language, with the other always replying in another language. Thus a truly bilingual conversation can take place. This was the case with Armelle's parents – her father spoke French to his wife and she replied in Spanish. It may feel uncomfortable at first, and in our experience it is quite unusual (we only found one example). But it can be an ideal solution in some mixed-language families and it is worth giving it a go. It does mean that the child hears speech in both languages that is directed at adults, and which is therefore likely to be much more complex and broad than the speech generally directed at children.

(C) Consistency in languages used to children / changing the language you speak to your child(ren)

(C 1) We think that it is probably easier for children, particularly when they are very young, if they hear one language at a time (i.e. complete sentences in each language), rather than two languages constantly mixed together. (This is not a problem if you both consistently speak your own language but alternately as just described above.) If you can easily separate out the languages, then we would say do so. But if you cannot, do not assume that you should give up or get very downhearted because of this. Several of our interviewees were surrounded by mixed languages but still easily sorted this out (e.g. Markus). If you do mix languages with your children, it probably helps if they also regularly spend some significant time with monolingual speakers so that they also acquire the habit of speaking each language without mixing (for Parvati this was achieved with monolingual child carers in her minority language, and Markus attended both German and English-medium schools). If they know that everyone around them is bilingual and can understand both languages, then it is very easy for them to mix languages a lot of the time. This is not a problem, so long as, when it comes to monolingual speakers, they can stop mixing and still produce fluent and rich sentences. Of course if you are the child's only source of input in one language and you start using words from the majority language in your speech, then you are pushing the input in the minority language still lower, and this would be a different case where mixing would also mean a reduced input in what may be a child's weaker language, and it is the reduced input which might have an impact on the outcome. Although you might think that the amount of the majority language may be very small (at first), it seems that this can be a slippery slope and in some families it can quite quickly result in an almost total switch to the majority language.

(C 2) What should you do if your children reply to you in only one (usually stronger) language, regardless of any rules you have tried to establish? As usual, it is complex but at the very least we can say 'Don't panic!' At least three interviewees had periods when they were monolingual when they were very small (Daniela, Ingrid and Astrid) which can be very worrying for parents when they have never heard their children say a complete sentence in one of their languages. However, these phases normally pass fairly rapidly. If your child speaks one language at home and another in the community and the child only speaks the home language, this problem will be solved when he or she starts nursery or school. If you are in a mixed-language family and the child is refusing to speak the minority language read the section of this book on resistance (Chapter 11). Try arranging a holiday for as long as you can possibly spare to a country where that language is the majority language. If this is not possible then see if you can find a Saturday school or preschool group where that language is spoken. It does seem to be important that your child is aware that you have a preference for them to speak the language that they are not replying in. This does not mean that you need to put them under pressure to do so or make them feel guilty for not doing so, but if you convey to your child that the language is not important to you, then this might affect their ability or willingness to speak it later.

Whatever you do, do not give up speaking the language to the child just because they reply in another language, this is almost certainly just a phase and, even if it may turn out to be an extremely long phase, most children do get past it. Resistance at slightly older ages is less worrying because it is often resistance to speak a language to a particular person or at home, whereas the child will speak that language when they need to (e.g. in a class at school, with other relatives or whilst on holiday). Certainly all those interviewees in our sample who resisted speaking a language over long periods, *provided that their parents continued to address them in that language,* ended up actively speaking that language fluently as adults. In two cases where the interviewees clearly understood that another language was equally acceptable to their parent, who may even have also switched to speaking another language to them, the final outcome in terms of language fluency (and usage) was less successful.

So at the very least your children do really need to know from you that you value a particularly language. If children will not speak it to you but speak it whilst on holiday, you could perhaps particularly praise this, and make clear how proud you are that they can do so. Some interviewees who resisted felt that their parents should have pushed them more. Others were grateful that their parents had not pushed them. If you can arrange for a holiday in a monolingual environment, where they will need to use their weaker language with family or in order to play with other children on the beach, in the campsite or around a swimming pool, this can help to at least reassure you that they can still speak the language when they choose to do so. And it will give them good practice in terms of actively speaking rather than simply passively understanding. Again, even if reading and writing is not a high priority for you, Saturday language schools provide an environment where children need to speak in a particular language in order to participate. It also gives them a peer group who speak that language which may tackle one of the factors contributing to resistance.

(C 3) How should you react if children start to gradually slip more and more words from their stronger language into sentences in their weaker language? Again there are very mixed views. In one case, where a parent insisted that a child spoke exclusively in a minority language when she started mixing the majority language into her sentences, the child resented the parent's insistence at the time, but she complied and this did not affect the outcome (although it might have subtly affected their relationship – this was the case with Josune, see p.67). Others recalled and valued their parents' clear expectations that only one language would be used at home whilst others valued their parents' flexibility. Some parents genuinely did not understand the majority language. Others, at times, claimed not to understand the majority language. Some parents ask the child 'What's the word in Urdu for ... [the word that the child had said in the majority language]?' And when the child supplies the word – which more often than not they did, in fact, know – will repeat the sentence back or ask the child to repeat the whole sentence in Urdu. Other parents supplied the word in the weaker language that the child had not been able to remember or produce.

One piece of advice is that if you do want to stop this, do not let a habit get established and then try to change it – you will need to address it right from the beginning. Antony and his sisters started speaking more and more English at home after they started school. Initially his father said nothing but eventually he decided that they should be speaking Greek. However the children's language habits were very well established, and he did not manage to get them to change back to speaking more Greek amongst themselves.

(C 4) It is probably not generally a good idea to change the language that you speak to your children whilst they are learning to talk – if you are tempted to do so, we would suggest that you wait a while as it is almost certainly better overall to make these changes later. In our experience, backed up by the interviewees' experiences, once children can talk quite fluently in either language, and particularly once they are aware that there are two languages involved (e.g. if they will say sentences like 'You speak English but my Baba speaks Kurdish' or 'Lola doesn't speak French'), it is less likely to cause a problem. We know of several families (interviewees and beyond) where parents have made changes once the children are past the first learning stages with no apparent ill effects, provided that the changes were made to rebalance the input, support or boost a weaker language, rather than to slide towards a majority language. The better reasons some gave for having changed were where parents who changed a language because they did not realise how imbalanced their children's input would be, and they wanted the child to get more input in the language which is not the community and school language, and which is usually the child's weaker language. Other parents have changed languages because their situation has changed (e.g. they have moved country) and what was once the majority language has become the minority language and, they feel, needs more support. However, be aware that these changes are often not at all popular with the children involved who will frequently notice and comment. If you are a family which has been operating a very fixed rule about who speaks what language or what language is spoken in a particular place, then it is likely to be quite a lot harder to change the rules (and keep to new rules) than if you have been a more relaxed family all along. Also, the older the children are and the more established the family's language habits, the harder it will be to make changes – particularly in the direction of a weaker and non-majority language.

(D) Try to make language either natural or great fun – certainly not a chore, use every resource at your disposal

As Josune has done, go out of your way to make associations between fun and your children's weaker language. If your child loves a particular character (Bob the Builder, Winnie the Pooh, Asterix, Tintin), see if you can find books or videos in your language featuring that character. If your child loves playing on the computer, see if you can find online games in that language. Clearly this is easier with national languages, and harder with marginalised languages. If you have a group of friends who speak a language you can meet up and do a favourite activity (from swimming to visiting museums or even eating out) with that group of people speaking a particular language. And so on.

Try to convey to your children that you value the language, which may also mean speaking positively about countries or cultures that use the language as a majority language. If your children hear you being critical of aspects of life in the countries where your minority language is spoken, try to balance this with celebrations of cultural events, lovely food, and so on.

(E) Starting mainstream school/changing the language of education

(E 1) If your children are starting school in the very early years in a language you do not speak at home, particularly if the school language is the language spoken in the community, do not worry at all. The fear that children in this situation will be disadvantaged, will fall behind and never catch up is a very common reason, in our experience, for parents deciding not to raise their children bilingually, which is very sad as it is based on a complete myth. Unless they have moved recently from another country, almost all of these children will, in fact, have picked up enough of the majority language from the community to understand a great deal of what goes on in a nursery or reception classroom. There may be some frustration when they do not understand everything or cannot necessarily say everything that they would like to say back to the teaching staff, but in our group these experiences were very rare and were always very short lived. It is not uncommon for some children in this situation to have a silent period when they do not speak at all at school (although in fact none of our interviewees reported this). Within six months your child should not only be understanding everything but also speaking more and more – albeit at a level appropriate for a very young child. If the system where you live is flexible enough to allow your child to start one year early and repeat the first year, this can be good (Ingrid's mother arranged this in Sweden). Starting school can be scary for children and, for some children, the fact that they do not understand everything, and that the language used is not the reassuring language used by their parents, may make the experience slightly more scary, but again this is the exception rather than the rule. Attending a more informal preschool or playgroup where the child will hear and may start using the language prior to starting school or nursery may help with this. Generally making sure your child is enrolled in a nursery or preschool or playgroup, or that you meet up with the community and give your child the opportunity to hear the majority language that is also the school language, is also a good idea.

(E 2) Check that the school is giving out positive messages about bilingualism. Make sure that any name-calling or racism expressed amongst the children is challenged by the staff. Where bilingualism is the norm, this is less likely to be a problem. However, in mainly monolingual countries such as the UK, the United States and France, being bilingual is sometimes seen as abnormal (and problematic). In England, for example, the term 'bilingual children' is routinely used by school staff to refer to any children who do not have a comfortable working knowledge of English, rather than to refer to children who speak two languages. As we have seen, for children who moved after the age of seven, there can be some challenges – some extra work for staff and extra resources being made available to these children. This means that many school staff view bilingualism as being less than positive. Children in mixed-language families who have spoken two languages from the very early days can be lumped in with children who arrive in a school aged 10 able to neither understand nor speak the language used at school. The one example in our sample (Marion) where the interviewee felt that being bilingual had a negative impact on her early years at school was also one where racism amongst pupils was unchecked by staff, and where the interviewee felt that the teachers had a very negative view of her preferred language (Welsh). If you are worried, talk to your child's teacher or to the school's head teacher.

(E 3) If you want to move country and/or you want your child to move to a school using a language that is new to them after they are around seven years old, you need to make an extra effort to make sure that this does not negatively affect them in the longer term. If at all possible, as soon as you know you may be moving, try to get some lessons for your children in the language that they will need at school. After the move, arrange either with the school or outside school for the children to get more support in their first year or so. None of the interviewees in this situation in our sample had any significant extra help outside school, although in three cases they were very positive about the special support that they received within school (Mumtaz, Fatima, and Shadi).

Perhaps ironically, the interviewees who already knew a language at home but had not been schooled in it, and who moved to schools to where that was the medium, actually received more help and support outside of school than those who did not know the language at all. Several families found ways of easing transitions even when the child already knew the language to at least some extent. This varied from Matilde's mother's arranging for her child to stay with the French-speaking nuns in Zaire, to Claudia's family hiring a tutor to help with her German, to Isabelle and her brother's year-long stint in a bilingual school between her years in the French and American school systems. Several interviewees remembered maths being a high point for them during transitions because it did not involve so much language; however, do tell your children that different countries have different ways of both teaching and doing even basic maths so that they are not too surprised and confused. Even if your children have quite a good knowledge of the language learnt at home, you may want to try to find out what they will be covering at school and discuss these subjects at home, covering some of the basic vocabulary with them in advance.

(F) Should your child attend beginner level classes in a language they already speak fairly well?

There was a wide range of views on this. Some interviewees found these classes useful. Although they found them easy, they were not bored (Claudia, Helen). Some interviewees found that they were useful in learning how to read and write (Pedro), or in improving reading and written skills (Armelle). Others used them to learn more formal language (e.g. Christine learning High German as well as the dialect her mother and her family spoke). Some attempts were made by teachers to use interviewees that were already fluent in the language as a resource for others. Some of these were at least partly successful (e.g. Armelle, Christine), others were not (e.g. Daniela who definitely did not want to be the teacher's pet). However, some interviewees had much more negative experiences. Some were simply bored; some misbehaved and got told off because they were bored. Ingrid did not attend English classes and went off to listen to Swedish tapes – with no explanation given – leading her to conclude, as a child, that her Swedish must have been poor. Christopher was told to just sit at the back of the class and do his own thing. Interviewees who had learnt American spellings were told these were wrong as teachers were using spellings used in the UK (Ingrid), and interviewees who gave a (correct) explanation of a word from their general knowledge were told this was wrong as it was not the definition in the textbook (Helen). One child who corrected a teacher who made mistakes was excluded from the class (Isabelle). Not all of the negative experiences were amongst the older interviewees – indeed, Helen was one of our youngest interviewees and Isabelle is also relatively young, so these cannot be put down to poor educational practices in the 1950s or before.

So our advice would be: 'Do not assume your children will not gain anything from attending these classes, but watch them carefully'. Make sure the language teacher is aware in advance that your child already speaks (reads, writes) the language. If you can do so, meet directly with the language teacher and have a conversation with him or her in the language concerned. You may gain some insight into his or her character and you may well be able to assess his or her language skills. (Teachers whose language skills are weaker or who have lower confidence are mostly likely to feel threatened by fluent pupils who may show them up.) If you have concerns, some suggestions include seeing if the teacher can use your child as a resource in the lessons for others, asking the teacher to set your child more advanced work, arranging for your child to go and assist in another (younger) age group – they are less likely to be worried about being a teacher's pet if they are not with their own peers. Some schools even with quite small numbers of children speaking a language have managed to arrange for those children who already speak a language to go to a separate class and to have a different type of lesson.

(G) Saturday schools

Try to find a Saturday school. (In the UK you can search by language and region on this site: http://www.ourlanguages.org.uk/schools.) Outside the UK, embassies of countries that speak a language are often aware of groups and Saturday schools supporting that language. (If your language does not have an embassy – Kurdish, Basque, Welsh – you will have to rely on your contacts and network and/or search on the internet.) If there is no school, think about whether you could start one. (In the UK ContinYou (http://www.continyou.org.uk/) has a special section that supports people doing or wanting to do specifically this – see under supplementary schools.) Again embassies are often supportive of such initiatives and may provide some start-up funding.

Try to make sure that the Saturday school is a fun experience for your children as much as this is possible. This can be difficult as different countries have different learning styles and teachers in Saturday schools will often replicate the style that they were trained in. Parents often support this because this style is often the one used when they were at school. However, in countries where primary schooling is very informal and a lot of learning is through play, children will notice the difference if a Saturday school is much more formal, stricter and a lot less fun. Some children will react more negatively to this than others.

If your child attends Saturday School, do not let them drop out without good reason. All of our interviewees who attended Saturday schools reported that they would have preferred not to attend when they were children, but all of the interviewees who dropped out regretted this and wished that they had attended for longer. All of our interviewees who did not learn to read and write as children either arranged themselves to learn as adults or regretted never having learnt.

(H) Identity

This is a really complex area. You have one of four choices, some of which can be combined.

(1) Make sure that the children know what they belong to. Establish a very firm sense of belonging to something. There was a clear tendency amongst our interviewees to see themselves as different and for some this meant not fitting in. Many therefore seemed to believe that they must really belong in the 'other' country, only to go to that country as young adults and find that they were seen as even more different there.

(2) Raise your children to know that they are different but to be proud of it. Snjezana exemplifies this when she talks about how she explains it to her son (see p.168).

(3) Raise your children with the view that their identity includes every aspect of their heritage (i.e. they have a mixed or double heritage). They are a mixture of things or both or several things. You will also want them to be proud of this (both Mohammed and Kwesi were in this group).

(4) You can also raise your children to believe that belonging (at least in terms of nationality) may be a very overrated and soon to be outdated concept, and that it simply does not matter. (Several interviewees expressed these views.)

Several interviewees said to us that it was important that both parents in mixed relationships should be positive about both parts of their children's heritages, or that migrant parents should be positive about the culture of both the country that they have left and the one that they are now living in. It is not uncommon for us as adults to be critical of countries' progress, systems or policies. I wonder if, as we do, we can make sure that children are aware of the distinction between the government of a country and the cultural heritage of that country. Even where we may be critical of government decisions or certain practices, I would hope that there would be elements of the culture (e.g. everything from folktales, music, films, art, poetry, drama, literature, fashion, food etc.) that we value and are proud of. Shadi, the child of refugees from Iran, discusses this distinction and her parents' attempts to bring her up with it in some detail (see p.169).

(I) Be aware of pressures on teenagers' time.

Many monolinguals mistakenly assume or believe that bilinguals divide a fixed amount of brainpower devoted to language between two languages (i.e. that they need to squeeze two languages into the same space used for one – and thus that they never learn either language properly). Those who are better informed know that this is not the case: we all have large areas of our brain that are under-utilised and adding languages just means that we actually use a larger proportion of our brains. However, what *can* be limited for bilingual children, particularly as they get a little older, is the available time for learning languages. Where parents are seeking to raise their children able to read, write, sit exams and study at higher levels or work in two languages, this view of bilingualism may have more validity when solely applied to the fixed amount of time available to children – particularly teenagers – which needs to be divided between school and homework, other activities and leisure. Here, hard choices will need to be made. So children who may excel as athletes, ballet dancers or musicians may need to spend considerable time devoted to these areas if they want to aim for careers in these fields. Doing this and achieving a university-level standard in two separate languages *may* put untenable demands on their time (but not on their brains).

(J) Do not accept advice about bilingualism from those who do not have specific expertise or experience

Sadly, both among the interviewees in this book and within our group we have come across examples where professionals have given ill-informed advice on bilingualism. Medical training, as a rule, does not cover bilingualism! Your doctor probably knows less about it than you do – you have after all, by now, read all or at least parts of this book! Sadly, outside of very few places like Quebec and Wales, the same low-levels of knowledge may also be true of teachers and even health visitors (in the UK their training does cover bilingualism). If you are given advice about bilingualism by a professional, particularly if the advice is to give up speaking one language to your child(ren), ask if they have had special training on bilingual situations. Provided that your child does not have any disability or any significant behavioural issues and you are speaking a language you speak well or fluently to your child, think very carefully before following any advice that suggests that you should stop speaking the language that you have always spoken to your child. (Especially if the advice is to give up speaking a minority language – which is much more common than advice to give up speaking a majority language.) In many areas, one health visitor or speech therapist will have specialised in bilingualism and you can ask if you can speak to a specialist. If this does not exist, please email us at info@wfbilingual.org.uk and we will see if we can put you in touch with a specialist through our network of contacts. You can also use a variety of web forums to get some informal advice about your situation (for some examples see Chapter 31).

(K) Expect uneven progress and do not give up!

The most important advice we can give you is: 'Do not give up when things do not seem to be going well'. Even if your child is refusing to speak a language at all, if you continue to speak it to him or her, at the very least he or she will grow up with a passive knowledge of the language. As an adult it is quite easy to convert a passive knowledge of a language into an active knowledge, and it is certainly much easier than learning a language from scratch. If you at the same time continue to give him or her opportunities to speak the language, he or she may well surprise you one day by speaking it fluently.

If you embark on this project, be aware that this is a rollercoaster ride, with highs and lows (or even a blacked out ghost tunnel – the teenage years!). We know that our interviewees were not too nostalgic, as, when asked, most suggested specific aspects within their bilingual childhoods that they *would* change. But when times seem hard, remember that, at the end of the day, *not one of our bilingual adults, (no matter what difficulties they surmounted along the way – and these were many – directly or indirectly linked to their bilingualism) would have wished that their parents had decided not to raise them bilingually.* So, on bad days, when you get disheartened, remind yourself that they *will* thank you later on.

31 Suggested Reading

We have a library of around 20 books and can recommend books that cover a range of subjects – there is a full list on our website. To start with there are three which are excellent:

(1) Baker, C. (2007) *A Parents' and Teachers' Guide to Bilingualism*, Clevedon: Multilingual Matters.
   This is the best book by an academic or expert. It is written in the form of questions and answers, which are all listed in the contents, which means that you can just read the bits that are relevant to you.
(2) Kenner, C. (2004) *Becoming Biliterate: Young Children Learning Different Writing Systems*, Stoke on Trent, UK: Trentham Books.
   An accessible and inspiring book about children learning to read and write in different languages. The examples used are English children also learning Spanish, Arabic and Chinese. Thus covering different alphabets and a character-based language.
(3) Cunningham, U. and Andersson, S. (2004) *Growing Up with Two Languages: A Practical Guide*, New York: Routledge.
   This is a very accessible book based on the experience of a Swedish/English family living in Sweden (and written by the parents in this bilingual family). It covers many of the common issues and is very practical.

Websites

- http://www.wfbilingual.org.uk
  The website of Waltham Forest Bilingual Group, it includes some quick guidance for parents, a calendar of our drop-in events, workshops and speaker events, and lists of recommended books, some with reviews.
- http://www.multilingual-matters.com/
  Specialist publisher on multilingual issues – lots of good books to order on the subject.
- http://www.multilingualliving.com/
  A very good site with loads of material and constantly updated. Good forums. It is run from the United States so some local terminology creeps in, but most content is very interesting and relevant anyway.
- http://multilingualfamily.co.uk/
  This site aims to link up those speaking the same language who live in the same area. At the moment it mainly lists language Saturday schools and clubs by area.

- http://www.continyou.org.uk/content.php?CategoryID=631
  Language schools for children (Saturday schools). A very useful organisation is the 'Resource Unit' which exists to support people running Saturday supplementary language schools (now part of a wider educational initiative called Continyou). They maintain a list of all the schools serving all the language communities countrywide. They also run training for people wanting to set up a school or who are already teachers or on management committees. You can contact them on 020 7700 8189, or via info@resourceunit.com.
- http://www.ourlanguages.org.uk/schools
  This is a database of language schools in the UK. It includes both complementary/ Saturday schools and mainstream schools. It is searchable by language, area and other criteria.
- http://www.literacytrust.org.uk/talktoyourbaby/Bilingual.html
  This website has good advice and useful 'quick tips sheets' on bilingual families available in 10 languages from http://www.literacytrust.org.uk/talktoyourbaby/ quicktips.html/language
- www.bilingual-matters.org.uk
  This site is linked to a group of researchers at Edinburgh University. It provides some questions and answers, and the group is willing to give talks at local schools.
- http://www.bilingualforumireland.com/index.html
  This group covers Ireland and encourages the formation of language play groups which are then listed. The group has also given talks to the general public, to teachers and at conferences on non-academic aspects of bilingualism.
- http://bloggingonbilingualism.com/2010/02/04/bilingual-pre-teens/
  There are now many different blogs about different aspects of bilingualism. This one site lists many of them, as well as bilingual online stores, bilingual online resources and much more.
- http://babybilingual.blogspot.com
  A blog by a mother (and aunt) who speaks a non-native language to her children with lots of advice for those in this particular situation.
- http://www.lingo.org.au/
  A campaigning site based in Melbourne, Australia, with links to local groups.
- http://www.spanglishbaby.com/
  A US-based site focusing particularly on families using Spanish and English. Regularly updated and a nice 'Ask an Expert' section. It also contains links to useful blogs (e.g. on online resources in Spanish and English for language learning).

About Waltham Forest Bilingual Group and How This Project Got Started

This research project was initiated by members of Waltham Forest Bilingual Group (WFBG). WFBG is a local voluntary group that exists to support parents raising their children speaking more than one language. It is very small, has no office and no staff. It was established in 2003 by Ricky Lowes, an English woman married to a Kurdish man. She had a wide group of friends and when her son Dana was born in December 2000 she joined the local National Childbirth Trust.

She had already been struck by the numbers of mixed-language families that she knew or had come across, how little most of them knew or were able to find out about raising children bilingually, and how little support was available from people like health visitors and so on. The NCT offers a service whereby they put groups of women who have just had babies in touch so that they can meet up and give each other mutual support. Out of six families in the group that Ricky was put in touch with, four were mixed-language families.

Ricky decided that something needed to be done. Firstly, in around 2001, she wrote an article for the NCT magazine on bilingualism and as a result of this quite a lot of people got in touch with her. An email group emerged: members of this group started to email each other to ask questions or to tell others about things that they had found out or about useful resources. Some time later, in around early 2003, Ricky invited everyone round to her house to meet up for coffee, and as many as 25 people squeezed into Ricky's front room.

It became clear that the group could not carry on meeting in people's houses as there simply was not enough room. Ricky got some very useful advice from Voluntary Action Waltham Forest about establishing a group which had a constitution, and which could therefore raise small amounts of money and hire a room to meet in. Waltham Forest Bilingual Group was then formally created one evening in May 2003.

Since then, the group has invited a number of leading experts on bilingualism to talk to our members. We run monthly drop-in events. We have created a website. We put together a small library of materials and we lend books and DVDs on bilingualism to our members. We have also developed and run two workshops for members; one focuses on the issues that arise for parents of children up to the age of four and the second focuses on slightly older children. More recently we have run talks on how to work with your child's school around issues of bilingualism and have given presentations at major conferences about the work of the group.

During these workshops we repeated something one of our speakers had said to us: 'When your children are grown up, they will be glad that you made the effort to raise them bilingually'.

Colin Baker is a professor at the University of Bangor, and the author of several key books on bilingualism for both parents and academic audiences. He had been a constant and generous source of good advice to the group. We asked him (as we had before on other issues) whether a book existed that backed up this statement. We felt that a book that interviewed adults who had grown up bilingually and asked for their views on their experiences as children would be useful in encouraging parents. Colin told us that he was unaware of any such book, and suggested that we might like to take it on as a project. We discussed this with Multilingual Matters, who agreed with us that it sounded an interesting idea and said that they would, in principle, be interested in publishing such a book. We approached 'The Big Lottery's Awards for All' funding stream who agreed to give us a grant to carry out the interviews and analyse and write them up. This book is the result.

Methodology

Our intention was never to carry out scientific research or to provide definitive answers. The number of variables in multilingual families is huge and it is extremely hard to separate out the impact of different factors in terms of contributing to or determining outcomes. (Ideally researchers would do a 20-year-long, very detailed and complex research project that tracks families raising children bilingually, which identifies and measures every potential significant difference between them, scientifically measures the children's abilities in all languages at different stages and reports on which are likely to affect outcomes. This is not that research project!)

This book is not intended to be a contribution to the academic literature, although we hope that academics and students will still read it and gain insights from it. It does not use the terminology commonly adopted by those researching linguistics. There are no references to other linked research (although clearly many of the conclusions that we have reached from these interviews will relate to findings reported in academic journals or publications). This book should be accessible to all parents.

We did not have a random sample of interviewees. Initially we put out a call through our various networks and accepted all those who volunteered to be interviewed.

After completing around 25 interviews, we analysed the issues and contexts that we had covered and put out a more selective call for those who had had experiences who would fill gaps that we had not yet addressed. There is no doubt that our first 25 interviewees included many highly successful bilinguals, many of whom had had relatively privileged and untroubled childhoods.

These people were very happy to come forward and talk about their very positive experiences as bilingual children. Those whose early experiences were more mixed or which included divorce, death or ill-health of a parent were not always as keen to come forward, and in many cases we had to positively seek these out. In the end our sample was still not representative of the general population in several respects. We interviewed 30 women and 13 men, 12 or 29% of our interviewees had at least one parent who had been to university (which is much higher than the population in general), and 31 of our interviewees themselves were graduates (even more out of line with the population in general), with two more interviewees currently studying on a degree course at the time of their interview.

Our interviews were 'semi structured' in that we started out with a range of pre-set questions but allowed the interview to develop with lots of follow up questions depending on the answers to our basic questions. (The base questionnaire is included below as Annex 1.) We also asked each interviewee to complete a language self-assessment (Annex 2). This asked them to state how confident they would be completing a range of tasks in each of their languages. We are aware that this rating is very subjective – different people would give the same level of ability or fluency different ratings, but as all we were interested in was the comparison between the ratings in two or more languages, we hoped that the interviewees would at least be consistent in their self-assessment across their different languages. We did not formally assess anyone's level of language – if they said that they spoke it fluently, or wrote it without mistakes, or spoke with or without an accent we believed them. Initially, we were concerned that as we did not pre-select the interviews, many of the interviewees would cover similar material. However, we were very fortunate, as, although clearly there are issues or experiences that do come up again and again, almost all of the interviews also contained something interesting, moving and/or unique.

Initially, the only requirement that we made for interviewees was that they were adults (i.e. over 18 years old) and had spoken more than one language as a child. In fact, all the interviewees were functionally bilingual as adults in at least two languages. Some were very balanced bilinguals. Others felt that one language was much stronger than others. Some could not read and write at all in one of their languages. Several spoke, read and wrote three or even four languages fluently. Some, although bilingual, had lost potentially third or fourth languages along the way. In most cases we only interviewed one person in any family, although two of the interviewees are father and daughter. The contexts in which bilingualism occurred varied hugely – some were static contexts with national or regional languages. In some cases, these languages were vibrant and positively viewed (e.g. French in Canada), others were oppressed but resisting (e.g. Spanish in Texas), whereas others were languages that were very much at risk of disappearing (Occitan in south-west France). Some other examples involved children learning English or French as perceived high status and highly valued international languages. Unsurprisingly, the other contexts mainly involved either migration or mixed-language relationships (or both).

Annex 1 Base questionnaire

Questions

Can you summarise for me how it came about that you spoke more than one language as a child?

Follow up questions for whatever has not emerged, or is not clear

Basics about who spoke what

(1)   Which languages did you speak as a child? (Any particular dialects?)

(2)   Who spoke which language to you?

(3)   Did this change over time or stay the same throughout your childhood and adolescence?

(4)   Which languages were widely spoken in the community that you lived it at the time?

(5)   Did this change over time or stay the same throughout your childhood and adolescence?

(6)   If a migrant, document home (e.g. one person one language etc.) and community language patterns for each period in each country.

Period 1 from ... to	Country	At home	School	Community
E.g. 1981–1985 (age 10–14)	Brazil	English (father), German (mother)	English	Portuguese

(7)   Note changes of city, school, even if family members changed.

Feelings about languages/resistance/parental reactions

(8)   Were there ever moments when you were proud or happy that you spoke more than one language?

(9)   Were there ever moments when you wished (even if only for a moment) that you did not speak two/three languages?

(10)   Were there any times when speaking the language was particularly useful?

(11)   Were you happy to speak xxx at home? Was it ever a 'bone of contention'?

(12)   Did you ever go through phases when you refused to speak one language? If yes, do you remember any specific reason or feeling behind this? What did your parents do? How long did it last?

(13)   Were your parents consistent in which languages they spoke? Do you remember your reactions to this?

(14) Did both your parents understand both languages? If not, did you ever attempt to take advantage of this?

(15) Family dynamics – were there arguments over languages between parents? Between children and parents?

(16) Were you rewarded when you spoke either language?

(17) Were you aware of any particular feelings your parents had about either or both languages?

(18) Were you punished/was there disapproval if you did not speak xxx at home?

(19) Did you ever 'trade on' speaking xxx? Was it a bargaining chip between you and your parents?

Siblings/wider family/community organisations

(20) What languages did you speak with your siblings?

(21) Some people have told us about other influences that were important in their bilingual childhoods e.g. grandparents – was this a factor for you?

(22) How about other members of the extended family – aunts, uncles, cousins etc?

(23) What about the wider community? Friends? Friends of the family?

(24) What about community organisations, religious activities, or similar?

(25) How about a child carer? – nannies, au pairs, baby sitters?

(26) What about holidays?

(27) Was there any politics linked to your languages? (e.g. Kurdish was banned in public/at school?) Where the language is linked to a political viewpoint (e.g. Basque separatism, Irish or Welsh nationalism), were you aware of this and how did it impact on you?

Education etc.

(28) Did you ever go to a Saturday language school or similar?

(29) What about holiday clubs/camps?

(30) What about reading? Do you remember learning to read in either/both languages? Which came first? Were you ever confused about the different ways the languages were written/read? How long did this last?

(31) What about teachers? Were they aware of your home language? Do you remember them approving or disapproving?

(32) What about your peers at school? Were they aware of the languages you spoke at home? Were you different or normal? How did you feel about this?

(33) What language did parents use to help with your homework?

(34) What about language lessons in secondary school? Did you learn more languages or did you sit through basic lessons in a language in which you were already pretty fluent?

Outcomes/identity/the future

(35) How do feel now about the fact that you were raised bilingually?

(36) How much do you use your different languages? Who do you speak your various languages to now?

(37) Would you say you are a balanced bilingual?

(38) Do you have a noticeable accent in either/any of your languages?

(39) Do you use a different language in different parts of your life?

(40) Is the language pattern between you and your parents as a child that you described earlier still the same today?

(41) Do you find you behave differently depending on which language you are speaking? (If answer gives basic cultural differences e.g. differences in body language or customs associated with one language, ask for deeper differences.)

(42) Does this ever make you uncomfortable? What about when the two worlds overlap?

(43) If you had to choose an identity – not necessarily your nationality – what would it be? Which language community do you feel you belong to? Or do you belong to both ... or neither? Where do you feel you belong? What makes you what you are?

(44) Has being raised bilingually ... benefited you or have you lost out ... financially? .... Culturally? ... In terms of identity? ... Emotionally? ... In any other way?

(45) Are you raising your children bilingually? Would you raise any children you have in the future bilingually? Why?

(46) What advice would you give to a family just starting out to raise children bilingually?

(47) If there was one thing you could change about your own bilingual childhood, what would it be?

Any of the below not already covered.

Where Born:

Age:

Lived:

Interviewee's Languages:

Mother: mother tongue(s),   other languages,

level of education,   occupation

Father: mother tongue(s),   other languages,

level of education,   occupation

Languages of any other people living in the household

Sisters and brothers and differences in age/position in the family

Interviewee' s Occupation:

Interviewee's Education:

Annex 2 Language self-assessment form

WFBG Grown Up Bilinguals   Language self-assessment

This is not scientific but it is to give us an idea of how confident you feel about using the languages you learnt as a child in different settings.

Name ....   Date ....

Which languages did you speak as a child?

1 ....   2 ....

3 ....   4 ....

Thinking about the language you have put down as number 1, please indicate how confident you would be today that you could carry out the following tasks in that language without making mistakes.

1	Very confident	Quite confident	Not very confident	Not at all confident
Talking and listening with a member of your family				
Talking and listening with a friend or acquaintance socially				
Reading a personal letter				
Reading an official letter				
Talking to a professional (e.g. doctor or lawyer)				
Talking at work to a colleague				
Talking at work to a client/customer etc.				
Writing a personal letter				

Writing an official letter				
Writing a report at work or similar				
Making a speech (in a formal setting)				
Writing something to be published				

Now rate the language you have put down as number 2.

2	Very confident	Quite confident	Not very confident	Not at all confident
Talking and listening with a member of your family				
Talking and listening with a friend or acquaintance socially				
Reading a personal letter				
Reading an official letter				
Talking to a professional (e.g. doctor or lawyer)				
Talking at work to a colleague				
Talking at work to a client/customer etc.				
Writing a personal letter				
Writing an official letter				
Writing a report at work or similar				
Making a speech (in a formal setting)				
Writing something to be published				

3	Very confident	Quite confident	Not very confident	Not at all confident
Talking and listening with a member of your family				
Talking and listening with a friend or acquaintance socially				
Reading a personal letter				
Reading an official letter				
Talking to a professional (e.g. doctor or lawyer)				
Talking at work to a colleague				
Talking at work to a client/customer etc.				

Writing a personal letter				
Writing an official letter				
Writing a report at work or similar				
Making a speech (in a formal setting)				
Writing something to be published				

4	Very confident	Quite confident	Not very confident	Not at all confident
Talking and listening with a member of your family				
Talking and listening with a friend or acquaintance socially				
Reading a personal letter				
Reading an official letter				
Talking to a professional (e.g. doctor or lawyer)				
Talking at work to a colleague				
Talking at work to a client/customer etc.				
Writing a personal letter				
Writing an official letter				
Writing a report at work or similar				
Making a speech (in a formal setting)				
Writing something to be published				

Feel free to add any comments (either about your languages or about this exercise)

Annex 3

Child aged	Language A	Language B	Language C	
Total				

Glossary

Throughout the book we have tried to use everyday terms for concepts. We do not use linguistic research terms (e.g. diglossic, L1, L2). However, quite often a term that has an ordinary everyday meaning has a completely different meaning when used by professionals or academics. For example, professionals and academics use 'community language' to mean a language used by a small group of people (e.g. Italian in London) whereas we suspect that many others would take it to mean the opposite (i.e. the language most widely spoken in the community at large). For this reason, we have adopted the terms minority and majority language, even though we are aware that not everyone likes them – at least their meaning is clear.

Active knowledge   Ability to speak a language (as opposed to being able to understand but not speak it).

Bilingual: Able to function comfortably in more than one language in at least one setting for each language (e.g. school, home, work or similar). Although technically this term should be used to describe people who speak two languages only, we use it to include people who also speak three or four languages. This is partly because of the name of our group – we always mean bilingual to mean multilingual regardless of how many languages are involved.

Community language   See Minority Language entry in Glossary.

Immersion   Putting someone in an environment where only one language is understood or spoken, thus almost forcing them to listen to and try to speak it.

International school   Any school primarily catering for pupils who are not permanently based in the school's location, regardless of whether the school uses only one or several languages as the language medium.

Language medium   The language used to teach children during their ordinary lessons.

Majority language   The language most widely spoken in the local area (e.g. in shops, markets).

Marginalised language   A language which is (or has in living memory been) banned, a language where negative statements about its value are (or have been in living memory) prevalent or common in the media or in every day situations.

Minority language	A language spoken by only a few people in the local area (i.e. it would not normally be used in most shops).
Mixed-language relationship	A family where the two parents have different mother tongues or first languages.
Mixing languages	Starting a language in one language and inserting a word from another language (e.g. *'Can you please take the Mülleimer out?'*). We also use the same term if someone says a complete sentence in one language and then they switch to another language for the next sentence.
Monolingual	Able to speak or understand one language sufficiently well to be able to feel confident that they can operate in a particular context without difficulties. (NB. There is a large group of people who are neither monolingual or bilingual because they have some knowledge of a second language but not enough to count as bilingual. This is important as sometimes we will recommend that a child has contact with someone who is monolingual. Here we mean someone who can neither speak nor understand any of a language – which thus prevents a child from communicating with them in that language or adding words from that language in to sentences in another language.)
National language	A language which is linked to at least one nation state. Some languages (e.g. Kurdish) do not have a state to support them.
OPOL	One parent, one language, or one person, one language
Passive knowledge	Ability to understand a language (but not necessarily able to speak it).
Quadrilingual	Able to function comfortably in four languages (in at least one setting for each language, e.g. school, home, work or similar).
Saturday school	A school where children participate in activities in one of their languages (normally the language not spoken in the wider community and not the language they speak at school). Saturday schools vary between those that are very focused on formal learning and particularly learning to read and write, and others that include a wide variety of cultural activities including music and drama. These are normally held on a Saturday but sometimes they meet one day after school.
Supplementary school	See Saturday school above.
Trilingual	Able to function comfortably in three languages (in at least one setting for each language, e.g. school, home, work or similar).
Waltham Forest Bilingual Group (WFBG)	A small voluntary self-help group for multilingual families, based in North East London, UK.

Index